Neurology - Laboratory and Clinical Research Developments

Neuroscience Research Progress

research-

Neurology - Laboratory and Clinical Research Developments

A Clinical Guide to Cerebral Palsy
Fabrizio Stasolla (Editor)
2022. ISBN: 978-1-68507-815-7 (Hardcover)
2022. ISBN: 978-1-68507-896-6 (eBook)

Botulinum Toxin: Therapeutic Uses, Procedures and Efficacy
James C. Lark (Editor)
2022. ISBN: 978-1-68507-817-1 (Hardcover)
2022. ISBN: 978-1-68507-826-3 (eBook)

More information about this series can be found at
https://novapublishers.com/product-category/series/neurology-laboratory-and-clinical-research-developments/

Neuroscience Research Progress

An Insight into Neuromodulation: Current Trends and Future Challenges
Natalia Arias (Editor)
Ana María Jiménez García (Editor)
2024. ISBN: 979-8-89113-445-4 (Hardcover)
2024. ISBN: 979-8-89113-531-4 (eBook)

Dendritic Spines: An Update
Ignacio González-Burgos, PhD (Editor)
2023. ISBN: 979-8-89113-080-7 (Hardcover)
2023. ISBN: 979-8-89113-138-5 (eBook)

More information about this series can be found at
https://novapublishers.com/product-category/series/neuroscience
progress/

Mustafa Usanmaz
Editor

Central Nervous System Infections

nova
Medicine & Health
New York

https://doi.org/10.52305/GGLQ6201

NOTICE TO THE READER

The Publisher has taken reasonable care in the preparation of this book but makes no expressed or implied warranty of any kind and assumes no responsibility for any errors or omissions. No liability is assumed for incidental or consequential damages in connection with or arising out of information contained in this book. The Publisher shall not be liable for any special, consequential, or exemplary damages resulting, in whole or in part, from the readers' use of, or reliance upon, this material. Any parts of this book based on government reports are so indicated and copyright is claimed for those parts to the extent applicable to compilations of such works.

Independent verification should be sought for any data, advice or recommendations contained in this book. In addition, no responsibility is assumed by the Publisher for any injury and/or damage to persons or property arising from any methods, products, instructions, ideas or otherwise contained in this publication.

This publication is designed to provide accurate and authoritative information with regards to the subject matter covered herein. It is sold with the clear understanding that the Publisher is not engaged in rendering legal or any other professional services. If legal or any other expert assistance is required, the services of a competent person should be sought. FROM A DECLARATION OF PARTICIPANTS JOINTLY ADOPTED BY A COMMITTEE OF THE AMERICAN BAR ASSOCIATION AND A COMMITTEE OF PUBLISHERS.

Library of Congress Cataloging-in-Publication Data

ISBN: 979-8-89113-660-1 (Hardcover)
ISBN: 979-8-89113-759-2 (eBook)

Published by Nova Science Publishers, Inc. † New York

I dedicate this book to my beloved family, who have always been there for me, and to my wonderful friends, especially Dr. Kenan Demir, who have never withheld their support. Without you, this journey would not be the same. Endless thanks.

Contents

Preface

Central nervous system infections have been a major health problem throughout human history. Infections of central nervous system structures such as the brain, spinal cord and meninges can cause serious complications and can be life-threatening. Diagnosis and treatment may vary depending on the severity of the disease and the causative microorganism. Today, advanced diagnostic methods and effective antimicrobial drugs greatly assist in the diagnosis and treatment of central nervous system infections. However, early diagnosis and appropriate treatment can significantly affect the course of the disease.

To be successful in the fight against central nervous system infections, we must remember that a multidisciplinary approach is essential. Specialists from neurology, infectious diseases, microbiology, intensive care and many other fields collaborate to ensure holistic care of patients. This multidisciplinary approach results in success in the evaluation, treatment and rehabilitation of patients.

This book aims to provide an in-depth understanding of central nervous system infections. In addition to describing the infectious agents, symptoms, diagnostic methods and treatment options, it also provides important information on prevention and management of the disease. By bringing together the experience and knowledge of our experts, it aims to provide a comprehensive resource for readers from different specialties.

Mustafa Usanmaz, MD

Chapter 1

Cerebrospinal Fluid Physiology

Mustafa Can Güler*, MD, PhD
Department of Physiology, Faculty of Medicine, Atatürk University, Erzurum, Turkiye

Abstract

The human brain works like the engine of an automobile. It has a certain place in the body within the skull. This restricted area requires control of intracranial pressure and the movement of the brain, soft tissue to prevent blows and their possible effects. In addition, the brain needs a balance of nutrients and electrolytes to maintain its viability and functions. It is possible to say that a magic fluid may meet all these requirements. Cerebrospinal fluid supports the brain and spinal cord in various ways. The human brain floats in cerebrospinal fluid, which serves as a cushion and protects against blows. It slows the motion of the brain in case of any impact or movement of the skull. Cerebrospinal fluid also regulates the brain metabolism by supplying the required substances, such as nutrients and oxygen, and removing waste products. Besides, cerebrospinal fluid is essential to diagnose and evaluate numerous diseases. When considering these features of cerebrospinal fluid, it is vital to discuss its physiology. Characteristic properties, formation, circulation, distribution, absorption, and similar features constitute the main physiological roof of cerebrospinal fluid. Ultimately, we tried to mention the physiology of cerebrospinal fluid.

Keywords: brain, cerebrospinal fluid, physiology, spinal cord

---

* Corresponding Author's Email: mcanguler@yahoo.com.

In: Central Nervous System Infections
Editor: Mustafa Usanmaz
ISBN: 979-8-89113-660-1

Introduction

The human brain is given a wide variety of properties. It is the control center of the human body. Around these significant tasks, it always requires to be supported within the narrow lines. The fluid part of the brain performs these actions. Due to the restrictive structure of the skull, the amount of fluid housing in the brain is limited. About 1600–1700 ml can fit inside the entire cerebral cavity, which houses the brain and spinal cord. Cerebrospinal fluid (CSF) constitutes approximately 150 mL of this capacity (Hall & Hall, 2020). An adult brain is about 1300-1500 g. The CSF reduces the actual weight of the brain through its buoyancy effect and carries it as the sea carries a ship. CSF is a colorless fluid that fills the ventricles, subarachnoid space, and spinal cord. The volume of CSF is about 150 mL and is formed 500 mL/day mostly by the epithelial cells of the choroid plexus. Choroid plexuses are the main source of CSF formation. Three or four times a day, the CSF is renewed. The CSF regulates brain metabolism. It includes several components as a part of the supplementary system of the brain. CSF carries nutrients to the glial and neural cells and removes metabolic products. It also functions as a lymphatic system (Brinker et al., 2014).

Besides, it prevents mechanical injury of the brain. The brain floats in the CSF which serves as a cushion and prevents the brain from sputtering into the skull. Thus, a non-intense head blow moves the entire brain with the skull. The CSF also regulates intracranial pressure. In addition to these properties, the physiology of the CSF is critical for understanding various central nervous system (CNS) diseases. It can be used to diagnose a number of clinical conditions, including a wide range of clinical illnesses. Neoplastic and neurodegenerative processes, inflammatory and noninflammatory diseases can be confirmed by CSF examination.

Cerebrospinal Fluid Spaces

CSF is present in two primary locations: the intracranial space and the spinal cord. The brain has four ventricles, which are fluid-filled spaces. The ventricles are composed of lateral ventricles, third, and fourth ventricles. They communicate with each other, as well as with the subarachnoid space that surrounds the brain and spinal cord through openings. The lateral ventricles are positioned bilaterally in the cerebral hemispheres. Foramina of Monro (right and left) connect the lateral ventricles to the third ventricle. The third ventricle lies in the diencephalon. The aqueduct of Sylvius connects the third and fourth ventricles. The fourth ventricle is surrounded by the pons, medulla, and cerebellum. Foramina Luschka (left and right) and foramen Magendie are connected from the fourth ventricle to the subarachnoid space. CSF is produced and circulates in the ventricles through these openings, and then reaches the subarachnoid space.

Cerebrospinal Fluid Formation, Circulation, and Absorption

The ependyma is a simple cuboidal epithelium that is lined along the ventricle and the surface of the spinal cord. The ependyma differentiates into a complex villous structure called the choroid plexus in some areas. Each ventricle surface includes the choroid plexus. Most of the CSF is produced by choroid plexuses. The remaining part, a small amount of CSF is secreted by ventricle ependymal surfaces and arachnoidal membranes. The formation of CSF is about 0.3 mL/min or about 500 mL/day (Cserr, 1971). The choroid plexus secretes CSF into the ventricles. Sodium (Na+) ions are transported through the epithelial cells by active transport. Sodium–potassium ATPase pumps execute Na+ transport. The flow of positive Na+ ions pulls negative chloride (Cl-) ions concomitantly. These ions raise the CSF osmolarity, leading to osmosis. Besides, glucose, bicarbonate (HCO3), and potassium (K+) ions are also transferred into the ventricles. The levels of these substances may show differences when compared to plasma. Compared to plasma, CSF includes higher concentrations of magnesium, sodium, and chloride and lower concentrations of calcium, glucose, uric acid, proteins, and potassium. These values are helpful for the evaluation of various clinical conditions.

The choroid plexus of the lateral ventricle produces the main part of the ventricular CSF. The CSF passes to the third ventricle through the foramen of Monro. A trace of CSF is produced here, added to current CSF, and carried to the fourth ventricle through aqueduct of Sylvius. Minutes amount of CSF is also produced here and the whole fluid is transferred to the subarachnoid space through foramina Luschka and foramen Magendie. The ependymal cells propel the CSF from the ventricles toward the subarachnoid spaces. Cerebral artery pulses also contribute to CSF flow.

CSF circulates in the subarachnoid space after leaving the ventricles. The CSF is then reabsorbed into the venous system by arachnoid granulations, and the cycle begins again. Almost 90% of the CSF is reabsorbed by brain areas, whereas the remaining is by the spinal cord. The formation of CSF is almost constant and thus the amount of CSF mostly depends on the drainage capacity of the arachnoid villi. Thereby, the CSF volume-related CSF pressure is regulated by the arachnoid villi. The arachnoid villi are composed of arachnoid cells. They protrude from the subarachnoid space towards the venous sinus. The normal CSF pressure is about 10 mmHg during lying in a horizontal position. When there is a health condition, CSF pressure may alter and lead to various diseases. For example, infections, tumors, and hemorrhage may increase the CSF pressure. It is possible to measure the CSF pressure and examine the fluid content through a lumbar puncture in terms of searching pathologies. When the patient is lying on his\her side, a spinal needle is put into the lumbar spinal canal below the end of the cord, to lumbar 3 (L_3)-L_4 or L_4-L_5 vertebrae.

The microvilli of these choroid cells are connected to each other by tight junctions that separate the extracellular space from the ventricular space. This structure is called the blood-CSF barrier that controls the passage rate of CSF and solute into venous blood. It is permeable to oxygen (O_2), water (H_2O_2), carbon dioxide (CO_2), and many lipid-soluble substances, very few permeable to electrolytes, and not permeable to large molecules. The blood-CSF barrier hardly allows several large molecules to transfer from the blood into the CSF. Pinocytotic vesicles may carry CSF and some macromolecules from CSF to blood. Some nutrients and other substances, such as glucose and vitamins, are transported by capillary-glial complex systems.

Conclusion

Within a variety of activities, the human brain has a great capacity for receiving, considering, and responding to stimulations. Besides, neurohormonal functions are a part of its actions. The high intellectual functions of the cerebral cortex are also crucial for homeostasis and maintenance of viability. All these properties require constant and adequate support service for an excellent working ability. The fluid content of the brain meets this essential performance. Even though the CSF is composed a few mL amounts, it is sufficient to overcome the expected demands.

CSF is a natural pool of brain tissue in which it easily floats. The CSF regulates brain metabolism through providing nutrients, electrolytes, and other necessary substances. On the other hand, it removes waste products. The CSF is circulated regularly and thus it refreshes the subarachnoid space and parts continuously. CSF is also substantial in terms of evaluating various diseases. All these results bring us to a point, emphasizing the importance of CSF. Thereby, it is inevitable to learn and understand the physiology of CSF. The formation cites, the circulation route, distribution, and absorption are primary components of the physiological processes.

References

Brinker, T., Stopa, E., Morrison, J., & Klinge, P. (2014). A new look at cerebrospinal fluid circulation. *Fluids and Barriers of the CNS,* 11(1), 10. https://doi.org/10.1186/2045-8118-11-10.

Cserr, H. F. (1971). Physiology of the choroid plexus. *Physiol Rev, 51*(2), 273-311. https://doi.org/10.1152/physrev.1971.51.2.273.

Hall, J. E., & Hall, M. E. (2020). *Guyton and Hall Textbook of Medical Physiology E-Book.* https://books.google.co.id/books?id=H1rrDwAAQBAJ.

Chapter 2

Overview of Infectious Diseases of the Central Nervous System

Emine Sehmen[*], **MD**
Clinic of Infectious Diseases, Samsun Gazi State Hospital, Samsun, Turkiye

Abstract

Central nervous system (CNS) infections are extremely important because of their rapid progression, leading to mortality and leaving permanent neurological damage. Today, meningitis remains a global public health problem (WHO, 2023). Many different microorganisms, such as bacteria, viruses, fungi, protozoans, and helminths, can cause CNS infections. The clinic of CNS infections can be acute, subacute, or chronic depending on the microorganism of the agent and the place of the involvement. Depending on the involvement, it can occur in the form of encephalitis, meningitis, abscess, or subdural empyema. Cerebral infections are most often seen in the form of acute meningitis (Tunkel, 2010).

Keywords: central nervous system infections, meningitis, encephalitis

Introduction

CNS infections are severe infections caused by bacteria, viruses, fungi, protozoans, and helminths (WHO, 2023). The clinic of a patient varies depending on the virulence of the microorganism and the place of its

---

[*] Corresponding Author's Email: sehmene@gmail.com.

In: Central Nervous System Infections
Editor: Mustafa Usanmaz
ISBN: 979-8-89113-660-1

involvement in the CNS. Patients may usually have a high fever, headache, focal neurological deficit, change in state of consciousness, or loss of consciousness. Since CNS infections can progress rapidly and are a life-threatening disease, early diagnosis, and appropriate treatment are essential for the prognosis. It is one of the emergency cases of infectious diseases that are life-threatening and have high mortality.

Overview of Infections of the Central Nervous System

CNS infections are severe clinical cases caused by bacteria, viruses, fungi, protozoans, and sometimes helminths (WHO, 2023). CNS infections are seen in the following forms (Tunkel, 2010).

- Meningitis
- Encephalitis
- Focal CNS infections: Such as brain abscesses, subdural empyema, epidural empyema, etc.

Meningitis

Inflammation of the pia mater and arachnoid membrane surrounding the brain and spinal cord is called meningitis. It is an infection of the cerebrospinal fluid (CSF) located in the subarachnoid space and inside the ventricles. It is the most common form of CNS infection (Anderson, 1993; Tunkel, 2010). In acute meningitis, symptoms progress in a few hours to a few days. The most common agents of acute meningitis are viruses and bacteria (Tunkel, 2010). Meningitis is an essential health problem in the world despite effective antimicrobial treatments and vaccines, and it occurs at any age. Globally, the most common agents of meningitis are the following four microorganisms:

- Neisseria meningitidis (meningococcus)
- Streptococcus pneumoniae (pneumococcus)
- Haemophilus influenzae
- Streptococcus agalactiae (group B streptococcus)

These four bacteria are responsible for more than half of meningitis-related deaths in the world (WHO, 2023).

Risk Factors for Meningitis

The patient's age, pre-existing disease, recent head injury, brain surgery, and cerebrospinal cord shunt are extremely important. In addition to the fact that meningitis is observed in all age groups, children are the most at risk. Especially in sub-Saharan Africa, meningococcal and pneumococcal meningitis are observed more in the world. The risk is high for those who stay in public and crowded places such as military wards, student dormitories, and migrant camps. People with immune deficiencies such as HIV, those with low complement, people with immunosuppressed, and smokers are at-risk groups for meningitis (WHO, 2023).

The most important microorganisms in acute meningitis are bacteria and viruses. Sometimes meningitis clinics can be observed depending on non-infectious causes (Tunkel, 2010).

The causes of non-infectious meningitis are as follows (Tunkel, 2010; CDC, March 30, 2022):

- Cancers
- Systemic lupus erythematosus (lupus)
- Some medications
- Head injury and brain surgery

Clinical symptoms of acute meningitis are usually high fever, chills, headache, changes in state of consciousness, and signs of meningismus. Signs and symptoms may include as follows (CDC, July 15, 2021; Tunkel 2010):

- Fever
- Headache
- Stiff Neck
- Nausea, vomiting
- Skin Rashes
- Photophobia (eyes being more sensitive to light)
- Clouding of consciousness
- Diarrhea

Symptoms of meningitis in newborns and infants:

- Inactivity
- Irritability

- Vomiting
- Not to suck, not to eat
- Bulging fontanel
- Abnormal reflexes

The agent bacteria of meningitis: (CDC, July 15, 2021).
Some reasons for bacterial meningitis are more likely to affect certain age groups:

Newborns:

- Group B *Streptococcus,*
- *S. pneumoniae,*
- *L. monocytogenes,*
- *E. coli.*

Babies and toddlers:

- *S. pneumoniae,*
- *N. meningitidis,*
- *H. influenzae*,
- Group B *Streptococcus,*
- *M. tuberculosis*

Teenagers and young adults:

- *N. meningitidis,*
- *S. pneumoniae*

Older adults:

- *S. pneumoniae,*
- *N. meningitidis,*
- *H. influenzae*,
- Group B *Streptococcus,*
- *Listeria monocytogenes*

Viruses (CDC, May 25, 2021, Tunkel 2010):

- Enteroviruses
- Mumps virus
- Epstein-Barr virus
- HIV
- Measles virus
- Influenza virus
- Arboviruses such as the West Nile virus
- *Herpes simplex* viruses
- Lymphocytic choriomeningitis virus

Protozoans: *Naegleria fowleri, Angiostrongylus cantonensis*

Risk Factors for Viral Meningitis

People of all ages can have viral meningitis. Therefore, some people have a higher risk of developing the disease, for example:

- Children under 5 years of age
- People with weakened immune systems because of diseases, medications (such as chemotherapy), and a recent organ or bone marrow transplantation
- Infants under one month of age and people with weakened immune systems are also more likely to have serious diseases (CDC, May 25, 2021).

Common symptoms in infants

- Fever
- Restlessness
- Loss of appetite
- Drowsiness or difficulty getting up from sleep
- Lethargy

Common symptoms in children and adults

- Fever
- Headache
- Stiff neck

- Photophobia (eyes being more sensitive to light)
- Drowsiness or difficulty getting up from sleep
- Nausea
- Restlessness
- Vomiting
- Loss of appetite
- Lethargy

Most people with mild viral meningitis usually recover on their own in 7 to 10 days. If viruses such as the herpes virus and influenzae are agents, antiviral treatment may help. Hand hygiene is essential for protection, and sick children should not be sent to school. The vaccines for mumps, measles, chickenpox, and influenzae are protective (CDC, May 25, 2021).

The first symptoms of viral meningitis are similar to those of bacterial meningitis. Therefore, bacterial meningitis is usually severe and can cause serious complications such as brain damage, hearing loss, or learning disabilities (Tunkel, 2010).

Bacterial Meningitis

Most community-based bacterial meningitis begins with the colonization of the nasopharyngeal mucosa. The contamination of the microorganism spreads from person to person through droplets and secretions (Tunkel, 2010; WHO, 2023). Bacteremia occurs as a result of mucosal invasion. Group B streptococci are carried through the human intestine or vagina and are passed from mother to baby during delivery. Not every microorganism can cross the cerebrospinal cord barrier. Those with trauma and congenital anatomical anomalies are at high risk for meningitis. Patients with immunoglobulin deficiency and splenectomized are exposed to a risk of infections of encapsulated microorganisms such as pneumococcus and meningococcus. *Listeria* spp. and Gram-negative bacteria can enter the bloodstream through the gastrointestinal tract and cause meningitis (Bhimraj, 2012).

It is an agent for 70% of all meningitis cases in *Haemophilus influenzae, Neisseria meningitidis*, and *Streptococcus pneumoniae*. The most common meningitis agents in the newborn groups are other enteric bacilli, especially Escherichia coli, *Pseudomonas* spp. and Gram-negative bacilli, and group B streptococci (Anderson, 1993). 70% of meningitis cases occur in the childhood age group. In the childhood age group *Haemophilus influenzae Neisseria meningitidis*; in the adult age group *Streptococcus pneumoniae, Neisseria meningitidis*; in the advanced age group, Gram-negative bacilli and *Listeria spp* are observed more often as agents (Anderson, 1993; Tunkel, 2010). N. meningitidis that causes meningococcal meningitis can cause major outbreaks. There are 12 identified serotypes of N. meningitidis, and 6 of them (A, B, C, W, X, and Y) can cause outbreaks (E). Mortality in untreated bacterial meningitis is as high as 50%. Even if diagnosed and treated early, mortality may remain at 8-15%, and sequelae such as brain injury, hearing loss, and learning disabilities may remain at 10-20% of the living (Oordt-Speaks et al., 2018).

Streptococcus Pneumoniae

Streptococcus pneumoniae is the most common cause of invasive bacterial infection in young children. The mortality rate of pneumococcal meningitis in children is at least twice higher than the mortality rate of meningococcal meningitis, and its sequelae rate is also high. In the last century, the increase in antibiotic resistance of S. pneumoniae has been significant. In antimicrobial therapy, treatment should be arranged based on the antibiogram of the culture of CSF fluid in LP (Tzanakki and Mastrantonio, 2006).

Neisseriae Meningitidis

It causes sepsis and meningitis in healthy children and young adults (Tzanakaki and Mastrantonio, 2006; Zhang et al., 2016). Neisseriae meningitidis is important in terms of causing outbreaks (Zhang et al., 2016). Rates of meningococcal disease in the United States have declined since the 1990s and remain low. In total, approximately 375 cases of meningococcal disease were reported in 2019 (the incidence rate is 0.11 cases per 100,000 people). Anyone can have meningococcal disease, but the highest rates of the disease occur in children younger than 1 year, and the second peak occurs during adolescence. Among adolescents and young adults, those between the ages of 16 and 23 have the highest rates of meningococcal disease. Because of the risks of severe morbidity and death, effective antibiotics should be administered immediately to patients with suspected meningococcal disease. Additional treatment may be required to eliminate the nasopharyngeal carriage.

About 10 to 15 out of 100 people with meningococcal disease may die. No more than 1 in 5 survivors recover, leaving sequelae such as follows:

- Loss of limb(s)
- Deafness

- Nervous system problems
- Brain injury

Infection

People transmit meningococcal bacteria to others through respiratory and throat secretions during close or prolonged contact. Close and prolonged contact, such as kissing, sneezing, coughing, or close contact with an infected person, catalyzes the spread of the disease. The average incubation period is 4 days, but this period can vary between 2-10 days. People with meningococcal disease and people who carry bacteria asymptomatically in the nasopharynx can spread the bacterium. The bacteria can spread from the nasopharynx through the blood to the brain. Humans are the only hosts (WHO, 2023).

Risk Groups

The domestic population or close contacts of patients are at the highest risk of progression of meningococcal disease. Infants under the age of one, adolescents and young adults aged 16 to 23, and adults over 85 have higher rates of the disease than other age groups. However, cases are observed in all age groups (CDC, July 2021).

Prevention

Vaccination is the most effective method of prevention. Vaccines against meningococcus, pneumococcus, and haemophilus influenzae type b (Hib) can prevent the disease. Hand hygiene, avoiding close contact, and not using common personal items are essential (WHO, 2023). The Bacille Calmette-Guerin vaccine protects against tuberculosis, but it is not widely used in the United States (CDC, July 15, 2021).

The CDC recommends meningococcal vaccination for all adolescents. Additionally, the CDC recommends that clinicians vaccinate children and adults who are at high risk for meningococcal disease.

The WHO has developed a global route map to end meningitis in the world by 2030. There are 3 goals for the "world without meningitis," and these are:

1) Elimination of bacterial meningitis epidemics
2) Prevention of 50% of cases and 70% of deaths with vaccination
3) Improving the quality of life related to meningitis and reducing meningitis-related sequelae (WHO, 2023)

The CDC also recommends chemoprophylaxis for close contacts of patients with meningococcal disease, regardless of vaccination status (CDC, July 15, 2021).

Health care professionals who have contact with a patient with meningococcal meningitis should take chemoprophylaxis in the following cases: mouth-to-mouth resuscitation, orotracheal intubation, aspiration of the patient, performing a bottom of the eye examination without wearing a surgical mask. With chemoprophylaxis, transmission can be reduced by approximately 89% (Batista et al., 2017).

Medications Used in Chemoprophylaxis

Ripampicin: 20mg/kg/day in children, 600mg/day in adults orally for 2 days with 12-hour breaks

Ceftriaxone: 250mg in children, 125mg in children under 15 years of age, single dose intramuscularly (recommended for pregnant women)

Ciprofloxacin: 500mg oral single dose (not recommended for pregnant women and children under the age of 18 years)

Azithromycin: 10mg/kg, maximum 500mg single dose

Amebic Meningitis

Primary amebic meningoencephalitis related to Nagleria fowleri is rare but fatal. Between 1962 and 2021, 154 cases were reported in the United States and only three patients survived. This microorganism lives in warm water all over the world and is transmitted to people through the nose, but it does not live in salt water. It is transmitted from contaminated waters to humans. Symptoms begin one to 12 days after infection and are similar to those of bacterial meningitis. It is difficult to diagnose, and there are very few laboratories that can perform specific tests. The presence of swimming in dirty water in the patient's history should bring this to mind. Combinations containing amphotericin B, azithromycin, fluconazole, rifampin, miltefosine, and dexamethasone are used in treatment (CDC, August 12, 2022).

Subacute and Chronic Meningitis

In subacute and chronic meningitis, symptoms can last for weeks, months, or even years. Fever, headache, meningismus, and changes in consciousness may also be observed in these patients. In these patients, high fever is not at the forefront at the beginning, there are usually symptoms such as weakness and restlessness. The symptoms progress slowly. The agents are listed as follows:

- Tuberculosis
- Spirochetes (Treponema pallidum, Borrelia burgdorferi)
- Mushrooms (Cryptococcus neoformans, Coccidioides spp.)
- Brucella spp.

Cryptococcal meningitis should be considered in immunosuppressed patients and HIV patients. In these patients, symptoms that develop subacute such as headache, fever, meningismus, and signs of personality change that last for days and weeks, are observed (Tunkel, 2010).

Encephalitis

It is a condition that occurs with neurological symptoms as a result of brain tissue inflammation. Symptoms include fever, headache, and change of consciousness, which are similar to symptoms of meningitis. In encephalitis, a change in state of consciousness is observed at the beginning of the disease. Acute cognitive disorder, behavioral changes, focal neurological symptoms, and seizures can be observed. In most cases, meningeal irritation may progress and occur as meningoencephalitis. The microorganisms that cause encephalitis are usually viruses (Tunkel et al., 2008).

Causative viruses: (Tunkel et al., 2008):

- HSV
- VZV, CMV, HHV-6 à usually in immunosuppressive
- Arboviruses (WNV, etc.)
- Respiratory viruses
- HIVà May be present with encephalitis or may be present in the form of CD8 encephalitis (immune reconstruction) under treatment
- *Epstein Barr* virus
- Measles virus
- Influenzae virus
- Nipah virus
- West Nile virus
- Japanese encephalitis virus
- St. Luis encephalitis virus
- JC virus

Causes of encephalitis other than viruses

- *L. monocytogenes*à Rhombencephalitis
- Bartonella spp.
- Mycoplasma pneumonia
- Rickettsia
- Ehrlichia spp.
- Coxiella burnetii
- Spirochetes (Borrelia burgdorferi, Treponema pallidum)
- Toxoplasma gondii à In immunosuppressants
- Protozoa (N. fowleri, Acanthamoeba spp.)
- Funguses (Coccidioides species, Cryptococcus neoformans, Histoplasma capsulatum)
- Helminths

Patients have symptoms of headache, fever, and changes in consciousness. Because the cerebral cortex involves diffuse in encephalitis, changes in consciousness and coma may be observed early. Since there is involvement in the cerebral cortex, a change in consciousness is observed at the beginning of the disease. Other signs such as speech disorder, personality change, and neurological symptoms related to focal or diffuse involvement can be observed. Sometimes, a clinical case may progress in the form of meningoencephalitis (Tunkel, 2010).

Encephalitis is most often caused by viruses (Tunkel et al., 2008; Tunkel 2010). Herpes simplex virus infections of the CNS can most often cause focal neurological symptoms by involving the temporal lobe. These are symptoms such as personality change, changes in consciousness, clouding of consciousness, and focal neurological involvement such as dysphagia, weakness, and paranesthesia may be observed. Arboviruses can be seen in summer and autumn, and Herpes simplex virus and HIV can be seen as sporadic cases throughout the year (Tunkel, 2010).

In an approach to the patient with encephalitis, an etiological diagnosis should be made. Although there is no specific treatment for most encephalitis, it is important from a public health point of view. The season of the disease, the region, the travel history, occupation, the insect sting history, and the status of vaccination are important in the etiological diagnosis. Examination of cerebrospinal fluid, blood tests, specific antibodies in the blood, and brain MRI should be performed in all patients. PCR testing in CSF samples is essential for diagnosis, especially in cases caused by herpes viruses. Electroencephalography (EEG) is rarely helpful in determining the etiology, but it should be performed on all patients with encephalitis. Brain biopsy should be considered in patients with encephalitis whose condition worsens despite acyclovir treatment in cases of unknown etiology. Acyclovir treatment should be performed in all cases of suspected encephalitis without the results of a diagnostic examination. In *Herpes simplex* encephalitis, early treatment of acyclovir is effective in reducing deaths and sequelae. Doxycycline should be started immediately when the rickettsial and ehrlichia agents are considered in the relevant season. Even though there are some studies indicating that acyclovir is slightly effective in varicella zoster encephalitis, the effectiveness of ganciclovir has been shown. It is recommended to use ganciclovir and foscarnet in combination in HIV-infected people (Tunkel et al., 2008).

Primary Amoebic Meningoencephalitis

They cause Naegleria fowleri, Acanthamoeba spp., and subacute granulomatous meningoencephalitis. These microorganisms live in the soil and are usually seen in the child age group as a result of playing in muddy water or swimming in a dirty pool. The amoeba passes from the nasal cavity to the nasal epithelium and spreads through the blood to the frontal and basal meninges, causing necrotizing inflammation. Symptoms appear 1-12 days after the infection. Patients have a serious picture of meningitis such as sudden fever and vomiting. With the appearance of symptoms, the disease progresses rapidly and usually results in death in 1-18 days, and mortality is high despite treatment. While in pleocytosis, in which polymorphonuclear leukocytes are dominated, high protein and a decrease in sugar are seen, Gram staining does not show bacteria in the examination of cerebrospinal fluid. During the recent examination of the CSF, mobile trophozoites can be shown under a microscope. In treatment, amphotericin B, azithromycin, fluconazole, ripampin, miltefosine combination, and dexamethasone are usually used (Anderson, 1993; CDC, August 12, 2022).

Neurobrucellosis

Brucellosis is the most common zoonosis in the world. *Brucella spp.,* which is an intracellular microorganism, rarely causes neurobrucellosis. It is transmitted through raw, not well-boiled milk, and dairy products. Headache, fever, weight loss, double vision, hearing loss, walking difficulties, polyneuropathy, depression, subdural hematoma, brain abscess, paraplegia may occur, and mortality is about 0.5% (Rose et al., 2009).

Tuberculous Meningitis

- Early/late complication of primary infection
- Basal meningitis, most often the 6th head pair is affected.
- Vascular changes; ischemia, infarcts
- Hydrocephalus (Anderson, 1993)

Diagnosis and Differential Diagnosis

Symptoms of meningeal irritation

- Stiff Neck – Kernig – Brudzinski
- Cranial nerve examination
- Lumbar puncture CSF sample
- A bottom-of-the-eye examination is required before LP.

Pathogenesis

The hematogenous pathway is the most important way for pathogens, including viruses, to reach the CNS.

In cases where the integrity of the dura is breakdown, bacteria can reach the CSF directly.

- Colonization and Invasion
- Intravascular survival
- Meningial invasion (Tunkel, 2010).

Focal CNS Infections

Brain abscesses, subdural empyema, and epidural abscess.

Brain Abscess

The local spread of sinusitis, otitis media, or mastoiditis to the brain, hematogenous spread, or trauma can cause the microorganism to reach the brain and cause infection. Headache, nausea, vomiting, and focal neurological symptoms can be observed. High fever is seen in less than 50% of cases. Aspergillus spp. and Mucorales can be observed in stroke cases. These microorganisms cause focal neurological symptoms due to their invasion of blood vessels. In patients with focal infection, back pain, radiculopathy, motor sensorineural symptoms, and even advanced paralysis can be observed as a result of spinal cord compression. If not treated immediately, neurological signs can be permanent (Tunkel, 2010). Parenchymal brain abscesses can be diagnosed by imaging techniques. A sample can be taken with a surgical operation, a microbiological diagnosis can be made, and successful treatment with effective antimicrobial agents can be performed (Anderson, 1993).

Subdural Empyema

It is an infection of the space between the dura and the arachnoid mater, usually caused by microorganisms spreading from the ear or nose. Rarely, it may also develop as the result of the hematogenous spread of a distant source of infection or penetrating head trauma. It can develop as a complication of meningitis in children. In adults with sinusitis and otitis, the agents are gram-negative microorganisms such as aerobic and anaerobic streptococci, staphylococci, *Pseudomonas spp.*, and Proteus spp. The most common agents in newborns and children are H. influenzae, Gram-negative bacteria, and pneumococci (Anderson, 1993). In the 10-year series of cases, French et al. reported that the most common agent of infection was neurosurgical procedures such as sinusitis, followed by chronic otitis media and mastoiditis at the end of ear surgery (French et al., 2014).

Clinical Signs

If there is fever, tachycardia, weakness, stiffness, sinusitis, or otitis, complaints related to them are observed. Headaches and meningeal irritation symptoms and vomiting, papilledema, and intracranial pressure increase-related symptoms may also be observed frequently. Focal symptoms such as hemiparesis, dysphagia, and less frequently cerebellar signs may be observed. Widespread or focal epileptic seizures may be observed. Imaging methods such as tomography and MRI are used in the diagnosis. MRI is a more sensitive imaging method in diagnosis. Appropriate antibiotics should be practiced immediately in the treatment. Anticonvulsive medications and intracranial pressure-reducing medications should be given prophylactically. Procedures such as burr hole aspiration and craniotomy can be required by neurosurgery. Early diagnosis, immediate practice of antimicrobial therapy, and surgical drainage are essential in reducing morbidity and mortality (Tunkel, 2010; Trench et al., 2014). In the study of French et al., for craniotomy to burr hole is recommended for surgical drainage at a more forefront level (French et al., 2014).

Diagnostic Methods for CNS Infections

In CNS infections, a lumbar puncture (LP) is performed, and a cerebrospinal fluid examination is the basis of the diagnosis. LP is the process of inserting a fine needle into the space between the 3rd and 4th or 4th and 5th lumbar vertebrae from the back under sterile conditions and collecting cerebrospinal fluid.

LP Contraindications

- Mass in the spinal or brain
- Infection of the skin in the puncture area
- INR>1.5 or platelet count <50000/ml
- Having used heparin in the last 24 hours
- Hemophilia and Von Willebrand disease
- Traumatic lumbar vertebrae
- Increase in intracranial pressure (Tunkel, 2010; Tunkel et al., 2004)

LP Complications

- Headache after LP (10-25%)
- Local bleeding (20%)
- Rarely infection (1/50,000)
- Back pain
- Implantation of epidermal tumor cells
- Post-puncture low CSF pressure syndrome
- Herniation (in the presence of a space-occupying lesion, intracranial pressure increase syndrome) (Tunkel, 2010; Tunkel et al., 2004)

Imagining before LP

- LP may be risky because of the cranial shift in cases where there is an intracranial space-occupying lesion such as cerebral abscess, or subdural empyema large infarct.

- The risk of cerebral herniation based on LP can be reduced with cranial imaging before LP.
- Imagings cause significant delays in starting the treatment. Who should get imagining before LP?
- The presence of focal neurological deficits (dilated unresponsive pupil, eye movement or visual field abnormalities, gaze paralysis, extremity involvements)
- New onset convulsive seizures
- Severe mental status change (GCS < 10)
- Severe immunodeficiency (organ transplant recipients and HIV-infected patients);

Besides these, there is no need for imaging before LP (Tunkel et al., 2004).

Examinations Carried out in CFS

The main methods of CSF are leukocyte count, erythrocyte count, glucose, protein, gram staining, and bacterial culture. Specific tests can also be practiced.

These are virus culture, tuberculosis culture, VDRL, ink pigmentation to examine cryptococcus meningitis, fungal culture, antibodies (IgM, IgG), PCR, and cytological examination (Table 1) (Tunkel, 2010).

Table 1. Cerebrospinal cord fluid examination findings according to meningitis agents (Tunkel, 2010)

Meningitis agents	White blood cell count (count of cells/ml)	Cell type	Glucose (mg/dl)	Protein (mg/dl)
Viral	50-1000	Mononuclear	>45	<200
Bacterial	1000-5000+	Neutrophils	<40	100-500
Tuberculosis	50-300	Mononuclear	<45	50-300
Cryptococcal	20-500	Mononuclear	<40	>45

Antimicrobial Treatment

According to the CSF examination, according to the agent it is essential to start appropriate antimicrobial treatment without delay. In this treatment, antimicrobial agents that are transmitted into the cerebrospinal fluid should be selected. Corticosteroids can be used in some cases to reduce meningeal irritation in treatment (Tunkel, 2010; Tunkel et al., 2004; CDC, July 15, 2021).

Surgical Treatment

In cases such as drainage of brain abscess, subdural empyema, and epidural abscess, antimicrobial therapy should be applied together with drainage (Tunkel, 2010).

Adjunctive Treatment

Morbidity and mortality are high in CNS infections. Other treatments may also be required because cerebral edema and intracranial pressure may increase in CNS infections. In this case, the most commonly used medications are corticosteroids. The practice of dexamethasone, from corticosteroids, immediately before the first dose of antimicrobial therapy helps to recover Haemophilus influenzae type b and pneumococcal meningitis in newborns and children, and pneumococcal meningitis in adults. Corticosteroids are effective in cases of cerebral edema, a brain abscess that has a mass effect on the brain. In the case of a convulsion, lorazepam or diazepam should be used. Patients with clouding or loss of consciousness should be fed intravenously and given liquid therapy (Tunkel, 2010; Tunkel et al., 2004).

Conclusion

The CNS can be infected with many microorganisms such as viruses, bacteria, fungi, and parasites. It can develop in the form of acute, subacute, and chronic infection depending on the virulence of the infectious agent, the place where it is involved, and the patient's immunity. CNS infections are important in terms of morbidity and mortality. Early diagnosis and treatment are the most important factors in reducing mortality and sequelae. Examining and determining the infectious agent is essential from the point of public health in order for the patient to receive appropriate treatment, as well as to protect the patient's relatives and prevent transmission.

References

Anderson, M. (1993). Management of cerebral infection. *Journal of Neurology, Neurosurgery, and Psychiatry*, 56(12), 1243. https://doi.org/10.1136/jnnp.56.12.1243.

Batista, R. S., Gomes, A. P., Gazineo, J. L. D., Miguel, P. S. B., Santana, L. A., Oliveira, L., & Geller, M. (2017). Meningococcal disease, a clinical and epidemiological review. *Asian Pacific Journal of Tropical Medicine*, 10(11), 1019-1029. https://doi.org/10.1016/j.apjtm.2017.10.004.

Bhimraj, A. (2012). Acute community-acquired bacterial meningitis in adults: an evidence-based review. *Cleveland Clinic Journal of Medicine*, 79(6), 393-400. https://doi.org/10.3949/ccjm.79gr.12003.

CDC (2022, August 12) https://www.cdc.gov/meningitidis/amebic.html.

CDC (2022, March30) https://www.cdc.tmlgov/meningitidis/bacterial.html.

CDC (2021, July 15). https://www.cdc.gov/meningitis/bacterial.html.

French, H., Schaefer, N., Keijzers, G., Barison, D., & Olson, S. (2014). Intracranial subdural empyema: a 10-year case series. *Ochsner Journal*, 14(2), 188-194.

Gul, H. C., Erdem, H., & Bek, S. (2009). Overview of neurobrucellosis: a pooled analysis of 187 cases. *International Journal of Infectious Diseases*, 13(6), e339-e343. https://doi.org/10.1016/i/ijid.2009.02.015.

Oordt-Speets, A. M., Bolijn, R., van Hoorn, R. C., Bhavsar, A., & Kyaw, M. H. (2018). Global etiology of bacterial meningitis: A review and meta-analysis. *PLoS ONE*, 13(6), 1-16. https://doi.org/10.1371/journal.pone.0198772.

World Health Organization. (2023, April 17). WHO meningitis key facts. https://www.who.int/newsroom/fact-sheets/detail/meningitis.

Tunkel, A. R. (2010). Approach to Patients with Central Nervous System Infection. In G. L. Mandell, J. E. Bennett, & R. Dolin (Eds.), *Mandell, Douglas and Bennett's Principles and Practice of Infectious Diseases* (pp. 1183-1188). Philadelphia, PA: Elsevier-Churchill Livingstone.

Tunkel, A. R., Glaser, C. A., Bloch, K. C., Sejvar, J. J., Marra, C. M., Roos, K. L., Hartman BJ, Kaplan SL, Scheld WM, & Whitley, R. J. (2008). The management of encephalitis: Clinical practice guidelines by the Infectious Diseases Society of America. *Clinical Infectious Diseases*, 47(3), 303-327. https://doi.org/10.1086/589747.

Tunkel, A. R., Hartman, B. J., Kaplan, S. L., Kaufman, B. A., Roos, K. L., Scheld, W. M., & Whitley, R. J. (2004). Practice guidelines for the management of bacterial meningitis. *Clinical Infectious Diseases*, 39(9), 1267-1284. https://academic.oup.com/cid/article/39/9/1267/402080.

Tzanakaki, G., & Mastrantonio, P. (2007). Aetiology of bacterial meningitis and resistance to antibiotics of causative pathogens in Europe and in the Mediterranean region. *International Journal of Antimicrobial Agents*, 29(6), 621-629.

Zhang, Y., Wei, D., Guo, X., Han, M., Yuan, L., & Kyaw, M. H. (2016). Burden of Neisseria meningitidis infections in China: A systematic review and meta-analysis. *Journal of Global Health*, 6(2). https://doi.org/10.7189/jogh.06.020409.

Chapter 3

Acute Bacterial Meningitis

Serhat Atalar*, MD
Department of Infectious Diseases and Clinical Microbiology, Ordu State Hospital, Ordu, Turkiye

Abstract

The main causes of community-acquired acute bacterial meningitis (ABM) are *Streptococcus pneumoniae*, *Neisseria meningitidis*, and *Listeria monocytogenes*, particularly in patients over 50 years of age or immunosuppressed patients. Staphylococci and aerobic Gram-negative bacilli represent the main causes of healthcare-associated bacterial meningitis. ABM should be suspected in adults presenting with fever and signs of meningeal inflammation. Even if patients do not present with the classic triad of fever, nuchal rigidity, and altered mental status, bacterial meningitis must be suspected in the presence of other symptoms attributable to the central nervous system (e.g., headache). ABM progresses with noise and quickly in a few hours. It is necessary to perform a lumbar puncture (LP) as soon as possible in all suspected meningitis cases unless there are contraindications, to determine the etiology, guide treatment decisions, and prevent unnecessary treatments and long hospital stays. Cranial imaging is not required in most cases prior to LP. Unnecessary imaging leads to delays in LP and antibiotherapy. In all patients with suspected ABM, a blood culture should be taken, a CSF examination should be performed with lumbar puncture, and CSF biochemistry should be studied. The isolation of a bacterial pathogen from CSF by culture or other diagnostic methods or growth in the blood culture of a patient with CSF pleocytosis without growth in the CSF culture confirms the diagnosis. Steroid therapy must

* Corresponding Author's Email: drserhatatalar@gmail.com.

In: Central Nervous System Infections
Editor: Mustafa Usanmaz
ISBN: 979-8-89113-660-1

be initiated with or just before antibiotic administration in all suspected cases of bacterial meningitis. Empirical treatment should be selected according to epidemiological risk factors and Gram stain results.

Keywords: acute bacterial meningitis, lumbar puncture, cerebrospinal fluid, pleocytosis

Introduction

Although meningitis or inflammation of the meninx is defined as an abnormal number of white blood cells in the cerebrospinal fluid (CSF), up to 8% of patients may not have CSF pleocytosis (Erdem et al., 2017). Acute meningitis represents a syndrome clinically characterized by the onset of meningeal symptoms within hours or a few days (less than 5 days). Acute meningitis constitutes 75% of all community-acquired meningitis cases, and unknown pathogens (the causative agent is undetectable in approximately 40%) and viral and bacterial organisms are its most common causes (Sulaiman et al., 2017; Ellis et al., 2022). Although subacute meningitis is often used for clinical manifestations longer than 5 days and chronic meningitis is used for clinical manifestations longer than 4 weeks, there is no consensus on this terminology. This paper will address acute bacterial meningitis (ABM).

Epidemiology

The incidence of bacterial meningitis in the US and Europe is 0.7-0.9/100,000 people. This rate is less than half considering the incidence of 3/100,000 people in the 70s and 80s. The incidence of Haemophilus influenzae type B, meningococcal, and pneumococcal meningitis has decreased in recent years after vaccinations (Hasbun et al., 2019; van de Beek et al., 2016). The incidence in Africa is 10-40/100,000 people (Brouwer et al., 2018). Despite the decreasing incidence, the possibility of encountering acute bacterial meningitis cases in clinical practice is high, and the prevalence of meningitis among emergency room visits is estimated to be 62-80 per 100,000 (Pajor et al., 2022; Hasbun, 2022).

Microbiology

ABM may be community-acquired or healthcare-associated. *Streptococcus pneumoniae*, *Neisseria meningitidis*, and *Listeria monocytogenes*, particularly in patients over 50 years of age or immunosuppressed patients, are among the causes of community-acquired ABM. Staphylococci and aerobic Gram-negative bacilli are usually among the causes of healthcare-associated ABM, depending on whether antimicrobial prophylaxis is applied prior to surgery and procedure (Hasbun et al., 2022).

In patients over 16 years of age, *S. pneumoniae* causes bacterial meningitis in 72%, while *N. meningitidis* causes bacterial meningitis in 11%. *Escherichia coli* and *Streptococcus agalactiae* cause about 35% of early-onset neonatal meningitis cases (Hasbun et al., 2022).

The risk of ABM is increased in patients with pneumonia, otitis media, mastoiditis, sinusitis, and endocarditis; various underlying conditions (e.g., splenectomy or asplenic conditions, multiple myeloma, hypogammaglobulinemia, alcoholism, malnutrition, chronic liver or kidney disease, malignancy, and diabetes mellitus) (Carter et al., 2022).

It has been associated with Listeria infections and the consumption of contaminated raw vegetables, fruits, milk, and cheese (Charlier et al., 2017).

Gram-negative bacilli (e.g., *Klebsiella* spp., *E. coli*, *Serratia marcescens*, *Pseudomonas aeruginosa*, *Acinetobacter* spp., and *Salmonella* spp.) have recently taken a more important place in the etiology of ABM. It is possible to detect these causative agents after head trauma or neurosurgical procedures, in neonates, older adults, immunosuppressed patients, and in the cerebrospinal fluid (CSF) of patients with Gram-negative sepsis (Tunkel et al., 2017).

Clinical Manifestations

Patients with acute bacterial meningitis usually present with a rapidly progressing and noisy clinical picture after the onset of symptoms. The classic triad of the disease consists of fever, nuchal rigidity, and usually changes in mental status with sudden onset. Nevertheless, all three features are not observed together in a considerable number of patients (Durand et al., 1993).

The common symptoms include headache (84%), >38°C fever (74%), altered mental state (71%), neck pain (74%), and nausea (62-74%). Less frequent symptoms include seizures (23%), aphasia or hemi/monoparesis

(22%), coma (13%), cranial nerve palsy (9%), rash (8%), and papilledema (4%) (Van de Beek et al., 2017; Hasbun et al., 2019).

It is possible to detect rashes, such as petechiae and purpura, in 11-26%. When detected, they are associated with 75-92% meningococcal meningitis. However, petechial rashes are not specific to meningococcus. Patients with Listeria meningitis may present with rhombencephalitis manifested by ataxia, cranial nerve palsy, and/or nystagmus (Bjilsma et al., 2016; Van De Beek et al., 2016).

Sinusitis or otitis (34%), pneumonia (9%), arthritis (7%), and endocarditis (1%) may be among the accompanying infections at the admission of patients with meningitis (Ellis et al., 2022; Hasbun, 2022).

During the physical examination, a decrease of 1-4 points in the Glasgow Coma Scale, fever >38°C, nuchal rigidity (30% sensitivity, 68% specificity), and Kernig (5-11% sensitivity, 95% specificity) and Brudzinski (5-9% sensitivity, 95% specificity) positivity can be detected (Thomas et al., 2002).

In laboratory evaluations, leukocytosis and elevated CRP levels are common, but low CRP levels can be detected in the early period. Leukopenia and thrombocytopenia are signs of a poor prognosis. Hyponatremia (30%) can be detected but is usually mild (Kornelisse et al., 1995). Since blood culture positivity (50-90%) is high in suspected ABM, at least 10 mL of blood cultures should be taken in two aerobic bottles with two separate interventions prior to antibiotic treatment. Nevertheless, the probability of growth in blood cultures taken will decrease after antibiotic administration (Tunkel et al., 2017).

Diagnosis

Of patients with bacterial meningitis, 95% have at least two symptoms of fever, headache, nuchal rigidity, or altered consciousness. However, these symptoms and signs may also be observed in other diagnoses (Khatib et al., 2017; Carter et al., 2022). Hence, meningitis should be considered in any patient presenting with two or more of these symptoms. Unless there are contraindications, LP must be performed to diagnose or exclude meningitis and determine its etiology. The CSF evaluation represents the first and most important examination for diagnosis.

Absolute contraindications to LP are conditions that may cause bleeding problems, such as increased intracranial pressure syndrome with the risk of cerebral herniation, thrombocytopenia, the ongoing use of anticoagulant therapy, and suspected spinal epidural abscess.

It is recommended to perform CT before LP in patients with one or more of the risk factors due to increased mortality and morbidity, depending on a loss of time and delay in treatment, unnecessary costs, and radiation exposure. CT can be considered before LP in patients with immunodeficiency (HIV, undergoing immunosuppressive therapy, transplantation, etc.), a history of central nervous system disease (mass lesion, paralysis, or focal infection), a new-onset seizure occurring within a week before admission, papilledema, an abnormal loss of consciousness, and a focal neurological deficit. CT is not recommended in patients without these indications since it has no clinical benefits and delays treatment (Park et al., 2022).

The isolation of a bacterial pathogen from CSF by culture or other diagnostic methods or growth in the blood culture of a patient with CSF pleocytosis without growth in the CSF culture confirms the diagnosis. While there are studies reporting a high CSF opening pressure with LP in ABM (mean 350 mm H_2O), there are also studies that report a wide pressure range (e.g., over 300 mm H_2O in 39% of patients, below 140 mm H_2O in 9% of patients) (Bijlsma et al., 2016; Durand et al., 1993).

Characteristic CSF findings in patients with ABM are white blood cell (WBC) count of 1000/microL and neutrophil percentage higher than 80%, protein above 200 mg/dL, glucose below 40 mg/dL, and CSF/serum glucose ratio of $\leq$0.4. Despite these typical CSF findings, the range of CSF values in ABM is very wide (Bijlsma et al., 2016; Durand et al., 1993; van de Beek et al., 2016). Table 1 contains the findings of the ABM CSF. Following traumatic LP, there may be a false CSF leukocyte elevation since both erythrocytes and leukocytes can enter the subarachnoid space. In such a case, "corrected CSF WBC" value formulations or automated programs can be used. In traumatic LP, approximately 500-1000 erythrocytes are counted against 1 leukocyte (Montes et al., 2019). The diagnostic accuracy of CSF lactate is better than CSF white blood cell count, glucose, and protein (Sakushima et al., 2011) in differentiating bacterial meningitis from aseptic meningitis, with 93-97% sensitivity and 94-96% specificity (Sakushima et al., 2011; Huy et al., 2010).

CSF culture represents the gold standard in the diagnosis of bacterial meningitis and is 80-90% positive in community-acquired diseases if the sample is taken prior to antimicrobial therapy. Multiplex PCR is a method that can be used to detect the most common microorganisms of bacterial meningitis in a single test and has sufficient sensitivity and excellent specificity. It is extremely beneficial in distinguishing between bacterial and aseptic meningitis and bacterial identification. Such tests can be conducted within 2 hours in most industrialized countries but are difficult to access due to the cost (Hasbun et al., 2019). Immunochromatographic tests (ICTs) can be used in such cases because they provide cheap and quick results. Although they have been originally developed for urine testing, ICTs have 94% sensitivity and 100% specificity in patients with proven *S. pneumoniae* meningitis. ICTs outperform CSF microscopy and culture in diagnosing or excluding *S. pneumoniae* meningitis, the most common ABM agent in adults (Ait-Ali et al., 2023).

Table 1. Typical cerebrospinal fluid findings in central nervous system infections (Hasbun et al., 2022)

		Possible	Less Possible
Glucose (mg/dL)	<10	Bacterial Meningitis	Tuberculous Meningitis Fungal Meningitis
	10-40	Bacterial Meningitis	Neurosyphilis Viral Meningitis
Protein (mg/dL)	100-500	Bacterial Meningitis	
	50-300	Viral Meningitis Neuroborreliosis Encephalitis Neurosyphilis Tuberculous Meningitis	Bacterial Meningitis (EP)
Leukocyte (cell/microL)	>1000	Bacterial Meningitis	Viral Meningitis
	100-1000	Bacterial Meningitis Viral Meningitis Tuberculous Meningitis	Encephalitis
	5-100	Bacterial Meningitis (ED) Viral Meningitis Neurosyphilis Tuberculous Meningitis	Encephalitis EP: Early Period

Treatment

ABM treatment must be initiated early and quickly. Blood cultures should be taken prior to treatment. When LP will be delayed or an etiologic agent cannot be detected in CSF microscopic examinations, empirical treatment should be selected considering age, risk factors, antibiotic use, and a history of allergy. A recent history of sinusitis, otitis, pneumonia (e.g., *S. pneumoniae*), recent use of antibiotics (e.g., drug-resistant *S. pneumoniae*), travels such as Hajj and Umrah visits (e.g., *N. meningitidis*), recent parenteral drug use (e.g., *Staphylococcus aureus*), progressive petechial or ecchymotic rash (e.g., *N. meningitidis*), a history of head trauma (e.g., *S. pneumoniae*), and HIV infection or other immunosuppressive conditions (e.g., *S. pneumoniae, Listeria monocytogenes*, *Cryptococcus neoformans*) are effective in determining empirical treatment. Since the risk of penicillin/cephalosporin cross-reactions with meropenem is 1% or less, it can be considered in patients with a history of anaphylaxis against penicillin. Although meropenem is effective against Listeria within the scope of empirical treatment, the treatment should be specific if there is Listeria growth in the culture. Table 2 contains empirical treatment recommendations in ABM according to patient age and specific predisposing condition.

In countries with ceftriaxone resistance rates higher than 1% for pneumococci, vancomycin is also recommended in addition to ceftriaxone for empirical treatment. Nevertheless, after pathogen susceptibility emerges, vancomycin can be discontinued according to the MIC value, and penicillin/ampicillin can be preferred (Tunkel et al., 2017).

Since the administration of dexamethasone prior to antibiotic therapy, especially in pneumococcal meningitis, reduces neurological sequelae, particularly hearing loss, it is recommended to be administered immediately before the treatment (10-20 minutes) or together with the first dose of antibiotics at a dose of 0.15 mg/kg or 10 mg every six hours. There is a disagreement between the guidelines concerning the initiation of dexamethasone, which has not been administered immediately before the antibiotic or with the first dose afterward. In the US, it is not recommended to initiate dexamethasone afterward if it has not been administered with or prior to the antibiotic. The European guidelines state that it can be initiated up to 4 hours after the antibiotic, with expert opinion. It is recommended that the initiated dexamethasone treatment be continued for 2-4 days at a dose of 0.15 mg/kg or 10 mg every 6 hours. It is appropriate to discontinue dexamethasone if pathogens other than pneumococci and H. influenzae grow in the culture (Ellis et al., 2022; Tunkel et al., 2004; van de Beek et al., 2016).

Ceftazidime, cefepime, or meropenem may be used for the empirical treatment of gram-negative meningitis. Colistin (usually formulated as colistimethate sodium) or polymyxin B should be preferred to meropenem if the organism is later found to be resistant to these cephalosporins and carbapenems. This treatment may also require intraventricular or intrathecal administration (Tunkel et al., 2017).

Table 2. Empirical treatment recommendations in ABM according to patient age and specific predisposing condition (Tunkel et al., 2004; van de Beek et al., 2016)

≤ 1 month	S. agalactiae, E. coli, L. monocytogenes	Ampicillin 75-100 mg/kg x 4 + Cefotaxime 50 mg/kg x4 OR Ampicillin 75-100 mg/kg x 4 + Gentamicin 5-7 mg/kg/day
1-23 months	S. pneumoniae, N. meningitidis, S.agalactiae, H. influenzae, E. coli	Vancomycin 45-60 mg/kg/day (divided into 3-4 doses) + Cefotaxime 2 g (every 4-6 hours) OR Ceftriaxone 2x2 g (*See the notes)
2-50 years	N. meningitidis, S. pneumoniae	
> 50 years	S. pneumoniae, N. meningitidis, L. monocytogenes, aerobic gram-negative bacilli	Vancomycin 45-60 mg/kg/day (divided into 3-4 doses) + Ampicillin 6x2 g + Cefotaxime 2 g (every 4-6 hours) OR Ceftriaxone 2x2 g
Basilar skull fracture	S. pneumoniae, H. influenzae, Group A beta-hemolytic streptococci	Vancomycin 45-60 mg/kg/day (divided into 3-4 doses) + Cefotaxime 2 g (every 4-6 hours OR Ceftriaxone 2x2 g
Penetrating trauma	S. aureus, coagulase-negative staphylococci (especially S. epidermidis), aerobic gram-negative bacilli (including Pseudomonas aeruginosa)	Vancomycin 45-60 mg/kg/day (divided into 3-4 doses) + Cefepime 3x2 g OR Vancomycin 45-60 mg/kg/day (divided into 3-4 doses) + Ceftazidime 3x2 g OR Vancomycin 45-60 mg/kg/day (divided into 3-4 doses) + Meropenem 3x2g
After neurosurgery	Aerobic Gram-negative bacilli (including P. aeruginosa, S. aureus, and coagulase-negative staphylococci (especially S. epidermidis)	
Immunodeficiency state	S. pneumoniae, N. meningitidis, L. monocytogenes, aerobic gram-negative bacilli (including P. aeruginosa)	Vancomycin 45-60 mg/kg/day (divided into 3-4 doses) + Ampicillin 6x2 g + Cefepime 3x2g OR Vancomycin 45-60 mg/kg/day (divided into 3-4 doses) + Meropenem 3x2g

The dosage recommendations are for patients with normal renal and hepatic functions.

*If dexamethasone has been administered, rifampin 1x600 mg can be added orally. If Listeria is suspected, ampicillin 6x2g can be added.

Prognosis

Whereas the case-mortality rate in adults is 16.4% and 8.9% in the 18-34 age group, it has been reported as 22.7% in patients aged ≥65 years (Thigpen et al., 2011). The mortality rate due to ABM can reach 54% in resource-poor countries (Hasbun et al., 2022).

ABM-related complications can be divided into systemic and neurological. Systemic complications, such as septic shock, DIC, ARDS, and septic arthritis, are usually the consequence of bacteremia, which frequently accompanies meningitis. Neurological complications, such as weakened mental functions, CRPS and brain edema, seizures, focal neurological deficits (e.g., cranial nerve palsy, hemiparesis), cerebrovascular abnormalities, sensorineural hearing loss, and hydrocephalus, may occur at a rate of 28%. Complications may develop at the time of diagnosis or during treatment. Delayed diagnosis and antibiotherapy increase the risk of complications (Hasbun et al., 2019).

Prevention

There are vaccines against S. pneumoniae, N. meningitides, and H. influenza, which are among the main causes of ABM. Vaccines against S. pneumoniae and N. meningitidis are recommended for adults with various infection risk factors. The routine vaccination of adults against H. influenzae type b is not recommended, except for individuals who have had a prior splenectomy.

There is no place for chemoprophylaxis for meningitis (e.g., pneumococcal) caused by pathogens other than meningococci and H. influenzae meningitis.

Conclusion

The co-existence of a few complaints of fever, headache, change in consciousness, neck pain/stiffness, and nausea is alarming for ABM. The LP and CSF examination should be performed in the early period for diagnosis or exclusion. It is recommended to perform CT before LP in patients with one or more of the risk factors due to increased mortality and morbidity, depending on a loss of time and delay in treatment, unnecessary costs, and radiation exposure. Since blood culture positivity (50-90%) is high in suspected ABM, at least 10 mL of blood cultures must definitely be taken in two aerobic bottles with two separate interventions prior to antibiotic treatment. Antibiotherapy should be initiated without delay. If LP cannot be performed or is delayed, empirical treatment with dexamethasone should be administered. Empirical treatment should be determined according to Gram staining and epidemiological risk factors.

Vaccine protocols should be promoted to reduce the disease risk.

References

Ait-Ali, Y., Bourlon, L., & Jacobs, F. M. (2023). Review of progress and challenges in bacterial meningitis. *JAMA*, *329*(16), 1406. https://doi.org/10.1001/jama.2023.2545.

Bijlsma, M. W., Brouwer, M. C., Kasanmoentalib, E. S., Kloek, A. T., Lucas, M. J., Tanck, M. W., van der Ende, A., & van de Beek, D. (2016). Community-acquired bacterial meningitis in adults in the Netherlands, 2006–14: a prospective cohort study. *The Lancet infectious diseases*, *16*(3), 339-347. https://doi.org/10.1016/S1473-3099(15)00430-2.

Brouwer, M. C., & van de Beek, D. (2018). Epidemiology of community-acquired bacterial meningitis. *Current Opinion in Infectious Diseases, 31*, 78–84. https://doi.org/10.1097/QCO.0000000000000417.

Carter, E., & McGill, F. (2022). The management of acute meningitis: An update. *Clinical Medicine, 22*(5), 396–400. https://doi.org/10.7861/clinmed.2022-cme-meningitis.

Charlier, C., Perrodeau, É., Leclercq, A., Cazenave, B., Pilmis, B., Henry, B., Lopes, A., Maury, M. M., Moura, A., Goffinet, F., Dieye, H. B., Thouvenot, P., Ungeheuer, M. N., Tourdjman, M., Goulet, V., de Valk, H., Lortholary, O., Ravaud, P., & Lecuit, M. (2017). Clinical features and prognostic factors of listeriosis: the MONALISA national prospective cohort study. *The Lancet Infectious Diseases*, *17*(5), 510-519. https://doi.org/10.1016/S1473-3099(16)30521-7.

Durand, M. L., Calderwood, S. B., Weber, D. J., Miller, S. I., Southwick, F. S., Caviness Jr, V. S., & Swartz, M. N. (1993). Acute bacterial meningitis in adults--A review of 493 episodes. *New England Journal of Medicine*, *328*(1), 21-28. https://doi.org/10.1056/NEJM199301073280104.

Ellis, J., Harvey, D., Defres, S., Chandna, A., MacLachlan, E., Solomon, T., Heyderman, R. S., & McGill, F. (2022). Clinical management of community-acquired meningitis in adults in the UK and Ireland in 2017: a retrospective cohort study on behalf of the National Infection Trainees Collaborative for Audit and Research (NITCAR). *BMJ open*, *12*(7), e062698. https://doi.org/10.1136/bmjopen-2022-062698.

Erdem, H., Ozturk-Engin, D., Cag, Y., Senbayrak, S., Inan, A., Kazak, E., Savasci, U., Elaldi, N., Vahaboglu, H., Hasbun, R. & ID-IRI study group. (2017). Central nervous system infections in the absence of cerebrospinal fluid pleocytosis. *International Journal of Infectious Diseases*, *65*, 107-109. https://doi.org/10.1016/j.ijid.2017.10.011

Hasbun, R. (2022). Progress and challenges in bacterial meningitis. *JAMA, 328*(21), 2147–2154. https://doi.org/10.1001/jama.2022.20521

Hasbun, R., Van De Beek, D., Brouwer, M. C., & Tunkel, A. R. (2019). Acute Meningitis. In *Mandell, Douglas, and Bennett's Principles and Practice of Infectious Diseases* (pp. 2948-2953). Elsevier Health Sciences.

Huy, N. T., Thao, N. T., Diep, D. T., Kikuchi, M., Zamora, J., & Hirayama, K. (2010). Cerebrospinal fluid lactate concentration to distinguish bacterial from aseptic meningitis: a systemic review and meta-analysis. *Critical care*, *14*(6), 1-15. https://doi.org/10.1186/cc9395.

Khatib, U., van de Beek, D., Lees, J. A., & Brouwer, M. C. (2017). Adults with suspected central nervous system infection: a prospective study of diagnostic accuracy. *Journal of Infection*, *74*(1), 1-9. https://doi.org/10.1016/j.jinf.2016.09.007.

Kornelisse, R. F., Westerbeek, C. M. L., Spoor, A. B., Van der Heijde, B., Spanjaard, L., Neijens, H. J., & De Groot, R. (1995). Pneumococcal meningitis in children: prognostic indicators and outcome. *Clinical infectious diseases*, *21*(6), 1390-1397.

Montes, K., Jenkinson, H., Habib, O. B., Esquenazi, Y., & Hasbun, R. (2019). Corrected white blood cell count, cell index, and validation of a clinical model for the diagnosis of health care-associated ventriculitis and meningitis in adults with intracranial hemorrhage. *Clinical Neurology and Neurosurgery*, *178*, 36-41. https://doi.org/10.1016/j.clineuro.2019.01.012.

Pajor, M. J., Long, B., Koyfman, A., & Liang, S. Y. (2023). High-risk and low prevalence diseases: Adult bacterial meningitis. *The American Journal of Emergency Medicine, 65*, 76–83. https://doi.org/10.1016/j.ajem.2022.12.042.

Park, N., Nigo, M., & Hasbun, R. (2022). Comparison of four international guidelines on the utility of cranial imaging before lumbar puncture in adults with bacterial meningitis. *Clinical Neuroradiology, 32*(3), 857–862. https://doi.org/10.1007/s00062-022-01143-4.

Sakushima, K., Hayashino, Y., Kawaguchi, T., Jackson, J. L., & Fukuhara, S. (2011). Diagnostic accuracy of cerebrospinal fluid lactate for differentiating bacterial meningitis from aseptic meningitis: a meta-analysis. *Journal of Infection*, *62*(4), 255-262. https://doi.org/10.1016/j.jinf.2011.02.010.

Sulaiman, T., Salazar, L., & Hasbun, R. (2017). Acute versus subacute community-acquired meningitis: analysis of 611 patients. *Medicine*, *96*(36). https://doi.org/10.1097/MD.0000000000007984.

Thigpen, M. C., Whitney, C. G., Messonnier, N. E., Zell, E. R., Lynfield, R., Hadler, J. L., arrison, L. H., Farley, M. M., Reingold, A., Bennett, N. M., Craig, A. S., Schaffner, W., Thomas, A., Lewis, M. M., Scallan, E., & Schuchat, A. (2011). Bacterial meningitis in the United States, 1998–2007. *New England Journal of Medicine*, *364*(21), 2016-2025.

Thomas, K. E., Hasbun, R., Jekel, J., & Quagliarello, V. J. (2002). The diagnostic accuracy of Kernig's sign, Brudzinski's sign, and nuchal rigidity in adults with suspected meningitis. *Clinical Infectious Diseases, 35*, 46. https://doi.org/10.1086/340979.

Tunkel, A. R., Hartman, B. J., Kaplan, S. L., Kaufman, B. A., Roos, K. L., Scheld, W. M., & Whitley, R. J. (2004). Practice guidelines for the management of bacterial meningitis. *Clinical infectious diseases*, *39*(9), 1267-1284. https://doi.org/10.1086/425368.

Tunkel, A. R., Hasbun, R., Bhimraj, A., Byers, K., Kaplan, S. L., Scheld, W. M., van de Beek, D., Bleck, T. P., Garton, H. J. L., & Zunt, J. R. (2017). 2017 Infectious Diseases Society of America's clinical practice guidelines for healthcare-associated ventriculitis and meningitis. *Clinical Infectious Diseases, 64*(6), e34-e65.

https://doi.org/
10.1093/cid/ciw861.

van de Beek, D., Brouwer, M., Hasbun, R., Koedel, U., Whitney, C. G., & Wijdicks, E. (2016). Community-acquired bacterial meningitis. *Nature reviews Disease primers*, *2*(1), 1-20.

van de Beek, D., Cabellos, C., Dzupova, O., Esposito, S., Klein, M., Kloek, A. T., Leib, S. L., Mourvillier, B., Ostergaard, C., Pagliano, P., Pfister, H. W., Read, R. C., Sipahi, O. R., & Brouwer, M. C. (2016). ESCMID guideline: diagnosis and treatment of acute bacterial meningitis. *Clinical microbiology and infection*, *22*, S37-S62.

Chapter 4

Aseptic and Viral Meningitis

Özge Kaya Korkmaz*, MD
and Havva Erdem, MD
Department of Pathology, Ordu University, Ordu, Turkiye

Abstract

Meningitis is an inflammatory reaction of the meninges. The term aseptic meningitis was coined by Wallgren in 1925 (Gard, 1954). Wallgren described aseptic meningitis in patients with acute onset of meningeal symptoms and sterile spinal fluid. The first published studies described this disease as a novel disease; however, Wallgren stated in 1951 that aseptic meningitis may result from a wide range of illnesses (Gard, 1954). The term aseptic meningitis refers to patients with clinical signs of meningeal inflammation with negative bacterial cultures (Parasuraman et al., 2001). The most common cause of aseptic meningitis is viruses (Desmond et al., 2006). We can evaluate non-infectious causes in three categories among the etiology of aseptic meningitis. These titles are respectively; systemic disease-associated aseptic meningitis, drug-associated aseptic meningitis, and neoplasia-associated aseptic meningitis (Tattevin et al., 2019).

A wide range of infectious and non-infectious factors are involved in the etiology of aseptic meningitis. Hence, a multidisciplinary approach should be adopted when discussing the clinical characteristics, etiology, treatment, and prognosis of aseptic meningitis.

Keywords: aseptic meningitis, viral meningitis, herpes simplex virus, drug-induced meningitis, neoplastic meningitis

---

* Corresponding Author's Email: balozge4@gmail.com.

In: Central Nervous System Infections
Editor: Mustafa Usanmaz
ISBN: 979-8-89113-660-1

Introduction

Aseptic meningitis is usually a non-bacterial, infectious, or non-infectious pathology of the meninges (Tattevin et al., 2019). Meningitis with an unknown etiology is described as idiopathic. Among infectious agents, enteroviruses (Coxsackie and ECHO viruses) account for more than half of cases, followed by herpes simplex virus-2, varicella-zoster, adenovirus, influenza virus, rhinovirus, mumps virus, HIV (Han et al., 2016). Non-infectious causes are discussed under three main headings, as systemic disease-associated aseptic meningitis, drug-associated aseptic meningitis, and neoplasia-associated aseptic meningitis (Tattevin et al., 2019).

Although viruses are most commonly responsible for aseptic meningitis, the term aseptic meningitis includes viral meningitis.

Although the etiology of meningitis differs, its symptoms overlap. Especially nuchal rigidity and related tests (Brudzinski and Kering tests) show positivity in these patients (Mehndiratta et al., 2012; Waghdharee et al., 2010). Patients with meningitis typically complain of fever, abdominal pain, nausea, and headache. Other symptoms of the disease include short and rapid breathing, loss of appetite, nuchal rigidity, and sensitivity to bright light (Kumar, 2005). Lumbar puncture and CSF collection are performed to identify etiologic agents.

Gram staining and CSF culture are negative in aseptic meningitis. In viral meningitis, white blood cell counts typically range from 80 to 100 cells/μl (pleocytosis) and a large proportion of lymphocytes (>80%) is present (Dumaidi & Al- Jawabreh, 2017). Pleocytosis is generally considered an important criterion in the diagnosis of viral meningitis.

Polymerase chain reaction (PCR) is the gold standard method for the diagnosis of viral meningitis. PCR detects viral DNA or RNA in the patient's CSF (Verstrepen et al., 2001).

Viral Meningitis

Enteroviral Meningitis

Enteroviruses are non-enveloped, single-stranded RNA viruses belonging to the Picornaviridae family. Based on molecular and serological characteristics, they are grouped into Enterovirus (EV)-A, EV-B, EV-C, and rhinoviruses (Pallansch et al., 2013).

Enterovirus-induced infections are mostly transmitted by fecal-oral or droplet transmission. Low socioeconomic status and poor sanitation are risk factors (Muehlenbachs et al., 2014).

Enteroviral meningitis is the most common cause of viral and therefore aseptic meningitis (Parasuraman et al., 2001). They often cause aseptic meningitis that occurs in late summer and fall (Kupila et al., 2006). The emerging signs and symptoms of enteroviral meningitis are not distinctive from other aseptic meningitis. The onset of symptoms typically includes headache, fever, vomiting, photophobia, and meningismus (Parasuraman et al., 2001). Meningitis caused by enteroviruses and encephalitis can sometimes have severe consequences. Poliovirus-induced infections may cause bulbar-spinal paralysis, resulting in respiratory failure in patients (Muehlenbachs et al., 2014). EV- 71 causes hand, foot, and mouth disease. Pulmonary edema and brain stem encephalitis can be detected in hand, foot, and mouth disease (Muehlenbachs et al., 2014).

The typical histopathological finding of aseptic meningitis is characterized by leptomeningitis with edema and lymphohistiocytic infiltration, sometimes accompanied by necrosis. Perivascular lymphocytic infiltration and occasional neutrophils may be observed in the parenchyma. Other findings include gliosis, microglial nodules, and neuronophagia (Muehlenbachs et al., 2014).

Immunohistochemistry can often be used to differentiate enteroviruses in pathology or autopsy specimens, but PCR is more reliable (Hsueh et al., 2000).

HIV Meningitis

Human immunodeficiency viruses (HIV) are one of the two types of Lentiviruses that infect humans, a subgroup of retroviruses, and over time cause acquired immunodeficiency syndrome (AIDS) (Weiss, 1993).

HIV is a neurotropic virus and causes various neurological diseases by affecting the entire central nervous system along the neuroaxis (Parry, 1988). In clinical series, neurologic complications are observed in 31-60% of AIDS patients (Post et al., 1988). The occurrence of neurologic complications is an indicator of a poor prognosis of the disease and is the second most common cause of death in AIDS patients (Boufassa et al., 1995). HIV often causes aseptic meningitis. As in other viral meningitis, patients present with a clinical manifestation consisting of fever, headache, and meningeal symptoms with sterile cerebrospinal fluid, mononuclear pleocytosis, and often normal glucose and protein levels. The virus is rarely isolated in CSF.

Patients infected with HIV can often develop secondary meningitis with other viruses and opportunistic microorganisms. Epstein-Barr virus, herpes simplex virus, cytomegalovirus, and hepatitis B are among the AIDS-related viruses that can cause aseptic meningitis. The most common fungal agents are cryptococcus, while Candida, Aspergillus, Mucor, and Nocardia are other fungal microorganisms that can be seen (Zunt, 2002). Toxoplasma, tuberculosis, and meningococcal meningitis are other reported agents. Neoplastic aseptic meningitis may also occur frequently in patients due to malignant transformation. Histopathological examination reveals perivascular mononuclear cell infiltrates, an inflammatory response accompanied by multinucleated giant cells and macrophages, and vasculitis areas causing axonal degeneration and demyelination (Santosh et al., 1998).

HSV Meningitis

Herpes simplex virus (HSV) can cause neonatal herpes in the central nervous system during the neonatal period, as well as herpes simplex encephalitis or aseptic meningitis, which has an extremely aggressive course, in children and adults (Tyler, 2004). While HSV-1 is responsible for 90% of herpes simplex encephalitis in adults, HSV-2 has been detected at a lower rate in patients. The majority of patients presenting with herpes simplex encephalitis have preexisting latent HSV-1 infection (Aurelius et al., 1993). Herpes simplex encephalitis has a very poor prognosis, resulting in death in 70% of untreated patients. HSV-2 is generally responsible for aseptic meningitis and recurrent lymphocytic meningitis (Tyler, 2004).

Recurrent meningitis (Mollaret's meningitis) is a rare disease characterized by three meningismus attacks within two to five days followed by spontaneous remission. HSV-2 is the most common etiologic agent in Mollaret meningitis (Marwan & Whitley, 2006; Tedder et al., 1994). In recurrent HSV meningitis, 40% of patients have a history of HSV-related genital lesions (Tyler, 2004).

The early diagnosis of HSE is of great importance for the rapid initiation of antiviral therapy to improve morbidity and mortality outcomes in HSV encephalitis. PCR analysis for HSV DNA in cerebrospinal fluid is recommended for the diagnosis of HSE. PCR has >95% sensitivity and specificity for HSV DNA in the first week after the start of therapy for patients with HSE. Although prophylactic use of acyclovir is not recommended, it may be considered in the treatment of very frequent recurrent meningitis (Tyler, 2004).

Diffuse edema and necrosis in the temporal and frontal lobes are among the histopathological findings of HSV infections. In the acute phase, meningeal and perivascular lymphocytic infiltrations, microglial nodules, and intranuclear inclusions are detected microscopically. Necrosis, neovascularization, and macrophage reactions are frequently observed in untreated patients. This, in turn, may lead to the development of atrophy and gliosis in the brain. Since inflammatory and reactive changes are more severe than other viral agents, they can be detected by imaging techniques.

Other Viral Meningitis

In the pathogenesis of viral meningitis, the etiological agent enters the gastrointestinal or respiratory tract through the droplet or fecal-oral route and causes primary infection. This is followed by a secondary infection of the central nervous system causing meningitis (Kohil et al., 2021). In addition to the viral agents specifically mentioned above, CMV, West Nile Virus, varicella-zoster virus (VZV), mumps, lymphocytic choriomeningitis virus (LCMV), EBV, and adenoviruses can also cause viral meningitis (Kupila et al., 2006).

Patients present with clinical manifestations such as headache, low-grade fever, and mild nuchal rigidity. PCR is often used for diagnosis. As with most other aseptic meningitis agents, it is characterized by mild to severe self-limiting inflammation. Histomorphological findings include lesions consisting of microglial nodules, lymphocytes, and macrophages. Necrosis may develop depending on the extent of inflammation. Cellular viral inclusions may be observed in some lesions.

Other Infectious Agent-Induced Aseptic Meningitis

Spirochetes: The spirochetes that cause aseptic meningitis are treponema pallidum and borrelia burgdorferi (Gray & Keohane, 2020).

Treponema pallidum causes syphilis and central nervous system involvement due to syphilis can be seen at any stage. However, neurosyphilis is usually observed in tertiary syphilis. HIV infection accelerates the development of neurosyphilis.

Lyme disease is a tick-borne multisystem disease that can cause meningitis, encephalomyelitis, and neuropathies in the central nervous system (Gray & Keohane, 2020).

Fungal infections: Central nervous system (CNS) fungal infections have high morbidity and mortality and have been increasing over the last three decades due to the high number of organ transplants, chemotherapy patients, intensive care unit admissions, immunocompromised patients, and hematologic malignancies (Nathan et al., 2021).

Two important fungal infections causing aseptic meningitis are cryptococcus and coccidioidomycosis. Organisms that infect humans through respiration then enter the central nervous system via the hematogenous route. Here, apart from meningitis, they can cause brain abscesses and granulomas.

Tuberculous meningitis: Tuberculous meningitis (TBM) may occur as the sole manifestation of tuberculosis or may be accompanied by pulmonary or other sites of extrapulmonary infection (Thwaites et al., 2009). Patients with TBM develop typical symptoms and signs of meningitis, such as headache, fever, and nuchal rigidity, although meningeal signs may be absent in the early stages (Chin, 2014).

In the evaluation of tuberculous meningitis, low glucose, high protein, and lymphocyte predominance are typically observed in the cerebrospinal fluid (Lee et al., 2018).

Anti-tuberculosis treatment should be started immediately and first-line anti-tuberculosis therapies have excellent CSF penetration (Slane & Unakal, 2022).

In tuberculous meningitis, it is very difficult to detect tubercle bacilli rapidly in the CSF. Hence, in regions with a high incidence of tuberculosis, tuberculosis should be considered in patients with aseptic meningitis. Clinical, microbiologic, and radiologic findings should be used together to support the diagnosis of TBM (Chin, 2014).

Systemic Disease-Induced Aseptic Meningitis

Sarcoidosis, Behçet's disease, Sjögren's syndrome, systemic lupus erythematosus, and Wegener's granulomatosis are the leading systemic diseases associated with aseptic meningitis. The diagnosis of meningitis caused by systemic diseases is quite challenging. Establishing this relationship can be clinically difficult. For this reason, the patient's history, physical examination, immunological tests, imaging techniques, and eye examination are necessary (Tattevin et al., 2019).

Sarcoidosis is a multisystemic disease characterized by the presence of multiple non-caseating granulomas (Vinas & Rengachary, 2001). Neurosarcoidosis is seen in 5% of these cases. Since the central nervous system is involved in patients with neurosarcoidosis; cranial nerve palsies, chronic meningitis, myelopathy-neuropathy, and neuropsychiatric symptoms are added to the clinic (Fritz et al., 2017).

Behçet's disease is a multisystemic disease that mostly affects young adults, although the age scale can be wide. Neurological symptoms in Behçet's disease usually appear as late findings. These include meningoencephalitis and cerebral vasculitis. In the differential diagnosis, the presence of neutrophils in the CSF is an important feature of Behçet's disease. The number of neutrophilic cells is usually >50 cells/mm3 (Tattevin et al., 2019).

Drug-Induced Aseptic Meningitis

Drug-induced meningitis is usually an aseptic meningitis with a diagnosis of exclusion and develops as an unusual side effect of medications. Non-steroidal anti-inflammatory drugs, certain antibiotics, intravenous immunoglobulins, intrathecal agents, and vaccines are some of the drugs reported as causative agents of aseptic meningitis. The CSF profile generally has a neutrophilic pleocytosis, and symptoms resolve several days after drug discontinuation (Jolles et al., 2000). Therefore, bacterial meningitis should be excluded from the differential diagnosis (Tattevin et al., 2019).

Neoplastic Meningitis

Neoplastic meningitis is a secondary inflammation of the leptomeninges characterized by tumor invasion. The diagnosis of neoplastic meningitis is made by identifying neoplastic cells in the CSF. It has been reported that 4-15% of patients with solid cancer and 5-15% of patients with hematologic malignancies develop aseptic meningitis during or after the diagnosis of neoplasia (Tattevin et al., 2019).

Although neoplastic meningitis has been described in almost all solid tumor types, the most common solid tumors causing neoplastic meningitis are breast cancer (43%), lung cancer (31%), and melanoma (6%) (Lombardi et al., 2011).

Patients with neoplastic meningitis present with rapidly progressive multifocal neurologic lesions, various motor and sensory defects, including cranial nerve palsies, and central and peripheral nervous system symptoms (Rigakos et al., 2017).

Lymphomatous meningitis in patients with non-Hodgkin lymphoma ranges between 1-20%. While CNS involvement is estimated to be less than 10% in adults with newly diagnosed acute lymphoblastic leukemia (ALL), the incidence may reach 12% in pediatric patients. Around 21% of patients with primary central nervous system lymphoma may also develop lymphomatous meningitis (Grewal et al., 2011).

Conclusion

Aseptic meningitis is a broad definition that includes many infectious and non-infectious diseases that cause infiltration of the meninges with negative bacterial culture in the CSF. Infectious causes of aseptic meningitis include viruses, fungi, spirochetes, and tubercle bacilli, while non-infectious causes include systemic inflammatory diseases, drug-induced and neoplastic meningitis.

The clinical presentation of aseptic meningitis is usually nonspecific, with fever, headache, nausea, photophobia, and nuchal rigidity being the most common symptoms. While bacterial culture and gram staining are negative in CSF analysis, pleocytosis $\geq$ 5 cells/mm ^{3} is detected. The biochemical examination of CSF usually reveals a normal glucose concentration and a protein concentration below 80-100 mg/dl. Nevertheless, the approach to patients with aseptic meningitis is complicated by the variety of etiologic agents and the relatively limited diagnostic tools available.

Viral meningitis is considered the most common cause of aseptic meningitis affecting different age groups. They often go unnoticed or lead to a self-limiting disease. Many viral causative agents such as enterovirus, parechovirus, and herpesviruses have been found to be associated with aseptic meningitis. In the CSF obtained for viral etiologies, virus-specific antigens, and PCR tests are usually performed.

The most common causes of systemic disease-associated aseptic meningitis are sarcoidosis and Behçet's disease. Solid and hematologic malignancies have also been found to frequently invade the central nervous system and cause aseptic meningitis.

The diagnosis of a patient with aseptic meningitis can be challenging due to the wide variety of etiologic agents, self-limiting viral diseases, and often a clinical presentation similar to that of bacterial meningitis. The history, physical examination, and cerebrospinal fluid findings of the patients should be well evaluated. Exposure to rodents, ticks (LCMV-Lyme), tuberculosis, previous primary viral infection, suspected sexual activity, systemic disease, and medication history should be questioned in the history.

It is necessary to make a diagnosis in a short time so that antimicrobial treatments related to the etiology can be administered urgently. In cases where bacterial-viral meningitis cannot be differentiated and culture results are not available, empirical antibiotic treatment is often initiated. Nevertheless, a rapid evaluation of a patient presenting with meningeal symptoms by a multidisciplinary team should be preferred to reduce mortality and morbidity and avoid unnecessary drug treatments.

References

Aurelius, E., Johansson, B., Sköldenberg, B., & Forsgren, M. (1993). Encephalitis in immunocompetent patients due to herpes simplex virus type 1 or 2 as determined by type-specific polymerase chain reaction and antibody assays of cerebrospinal fluid. *J Med Virol, 39*(3), 179-86. https://doi.org/10.1002/jmv.1890390302.

Boufassa, F., Bachmeyer, C., Carré, N., Deveau, C., Persoz, A., Jadand, C., Séréni, D., & Bucquet, D. (1995). Influence of neurologic manifestations of primary human immunodeficiency virus infection on disease progression. SEROCO Study Group. *J Infect Dis, 171*(5), 1190-5. https://doi.org/10.1093/infdis/171.5.1190.

Chin, J. H. (2014). Tuberculous meningitis: Diagnostic and therapeutic challenges. Neurol Clin Pract, 4(3), 199-205. https://doi.org/10.1212/CPJ.0000000000000023.

Desmond, R. A., Accortt, N. A., Talley, L., Villano, S. A., Soong, S. J., & Whitley, R. J. (2006). Enteroviral meningitis: natural history and outcome of pleconaril therapy. *Antimicrob Agents Chemother, 50*(7), 2409-14. https://doi.org/10.1128/AAC.00227-06.

Dumaidi, K., & Al-Jawabreh, A. (2017). Molecular detection and genotyping of enteroviruses from CSF samples of patients with suspected sepsis-like illness and/or aseptic meningitis from 2012 to 2015 in West Bank, Palestine. *PLoS One, 12*(2):e0172357. https://doi.org/10.1371/journal.pone.0172357.

Fritz, D., Voortman, M., van de Beek, D., Drent, M., & Brouwer, M.C. (2017). Many faces of neurosarcoidosis: from chronic meningitis to myelopathy. *Curr Opin Pulm Med, 23*(5), 439-446. https://doi.org/10.1097/MCP.0000000000000401.

Gard, S. (1954). The Etiology of Acute Aseptic Meningitis (Wallgren). *Acta Paediatrica, 43*(s100), 54–64. https://doi:10.1111/j.1651-2227.1954.tb15456.x.

Grewal, J., Saria, M., Grewal, H. K., & Kesari, S. (2011). Neoplastic meningitis resulting from hematological malignancies: pharmacokinetic considerations and maximizing outcome. *Clin Investig (Lond), 1*(10), 1391-1402. https://doi.org/10.4155/cli.11.115.

Gray, F., & Keohane, C. (2020). Spirochetal Infections of the CNS. In Infections ofthe Central Nervous System. In F. Chrétien, K. T., Wong, L. R., Sharer, C., Keohane and F. Gray (Eds.), *Infections of the Central Nervous System: Pathology and Genetics*. Wiley. https://doi.org/10.1002/9781119467748.ch38.

Han, S. H., Choi, H. Y., Kim, J. M., Park, K. R., Youn, Y. C., & Shin, H. W. (2016). Etiology of aseptic meningitis and clinical characteristics in immune-competent adults. *J Med Virol, 88*(1), 175-9. https://doi.org/10.1002/jmv.24316.

Hsueh, C., Jung, S. M., Shih, S. R., Kuo, T. T., Shieh, W. J., Zaki, S., Lin, T. Y., Chang, L. Y., Ning, H. C., & Yen, D. C. (2000). Acute encephalomyelitis during an outbreak of enterovirus type 71 infection in Taiwan: report of an autopsy case with pathologic, immunofluorescence, and molecular studies. *Mod Pathol, 13*(11), 1200-5. https://doi.org/10.1038/modpathol.3880222.

Jolles, S., Sewell, W. A., & Leighton, C. (2000). Drug-induced aseptic meningitis: diagnosis and management. *Drug Saf, 22*(3), 215-26. https://doi.org/10.2165/00002018-200022030- 00005.

Kohil, A., Jemmieh, S., Smatti, M. K., & Yassine, M. H. (2021). Viral meningitis: an overview. *Arch Virol, 166*, 335–345. https://doi.org/10.1007/s00705-020-04891-1.

Kumar, R. (2005). Aseptic meningitis: diagnosis and management. *Indian J Pediatr,* 72(1):57-63. https://doi: 10.1007/BF02760582.

Kupila, L., Vuorinen, T., Vainionpää, R., Hukkanen, V., Marttila, R. J., & Kotilainen, P. (2006). Etiology of aseptic meningitis and encephalitis in an adult population. *Neurology, 66*(1):75-80. https://doi.org/10.1212/01.wnl.0000191407.81333.00.

Lee, S. A., Kim, S. W., Chang, H. H., Jung, H., Kim, Y., Hwang, S., Kim, S., Park, H. K., & Lee, J. M. (2018). A New Scoring System for the Differential Diagnosis between Tuberculous Meningitis and Viral Meningitis. *J Korean Med Sci, 33*(31), e201. https://doi.org/10.3346/jkms.2018.33.e201.

Lombardi, G., Zustovich, F., Farina, P., Della Puppa, A., Manara, R., Cecchin, D., Brunello, A., Cappetta, A., & Zagonel, V. (2011). Neoplastic meningitis from solid tumors: new diagnostic and therapeutic approaches. *Oncologist, 16*(8), 1175-88. https://doi.org/10.1634/theoncologist.2011-0101.

Marwan, S., & Whitley, R. C. (2006). Recurrent Benign Lymphocytic Meningitis, *Clinical Infectious Diseases, 43*(9), 1194–1197. https://doi.org/10.1086/508281.

Mehndiratta, M., Nayak, R., Garg, H., Kumar, M., & Pandey, S. Appraisal of Kernig's and Brudzinski's sign in meningitis. (2012). *Ann Indian Acad Neurol, 15*(4), 287-8. https://doi.org/10.4103/0972-2327.104337.

Muehlenbachs, A., Bhatnagar, J., & Zaki, S. R. (2014). Tissue tropism, pathology and pathogenesis of enterovirus infection. *The Journal of Pathology, 235*(2), 217– 228. https://doi:10.1002/path.4438.

Nathan, C. L., Emmert, B. E., Nelson, E., & Berger, J. R. (2021). CNS fungal infections: A review. *J Neurol Sci, 422*:117325. https://doi.org/10.1016/j.jns.2021.117325.

Pallansch, M. A., Oberste, M. S., & Whitton, J. L. (2013). Enteroviruses: polioviruses, coxsackieviruses, echoviruses, and newer enteroviruses. In Fields, B. N., Knipe, D. M., Howley, P. M. (Eds), *Fields Virology* (6th ed., 490–530). Philadelphia, PA: Wolters Kluwer/Lippincott Williams & Wilkins Health.

Parasuraman, T. V., Frenia, K., & Romero, J. (2001). Enteroviral meningitis. Cost of illness and considerations for the economic evaluation of potential therapies. *Pharmacoeconomics, 19*(1), 3-12. https://doi.org/10.2165/00019053-200119010-00001.

Parry, G. J. (1988). Peripheral neuropathies associated with human immunodeficiency virus infection. *Annals of Neurology, 23*(S1), S49–S53. https://doi:10.1002/ana.410230714.

Post, M., Tate, L., Quencer, R., Hensley, G., Berger, Sheremata, W., & Maul, G. (1988). CT, MR, and pathology in HIV encephalitis and meningitis. *American Journal of Roentgenology, 151*(2), 373–380.

Rigakos, G., Liakou, C.I., Felipe, N., Orkoulas-Razis, D., & Razis, E. (2017). Clinical presentation, diagnosis, and radiological findings of neoplastic meningitis. *Cancer Control, 24*(1):9-21. https://doi.org/10.1177/107327481702400103.

Santosh, V., Yasha, T. C., Panda, K. M., Das, S., Satishchandra, P., Gourie-Devi, M., Ravi, V., Desai, A., Khanna, N., Chandramuki, A., Swamy, H. S., Nagaraja, D., Sastry, Kolluri V. R, & Shankar, S.K. (1998). Pathology of AIDS - Study from a Neuropsychiatry Centre from South India. *Annals of Indian Academy of Neurology, 1*(2), 71-82.

Slane, V. H., & Unakal, C. G. (2022). Tuberculous Meningitis. [Updated 2022 Nov 18]. In: *StatPearls [Internet]*. Treasure Island (FL): StatPearls Publishing; 2022 Jan-. Available from: https://www.ncbi.nlm.nih.gov/books/NBK541015/.

Tattevin, P., Tchamgoué, S., Belem, A., Bénézit, F., Pronier, C., & Revest, M. (2019). Aseptic meningitis. Revue Neurologique. *Rev Neurol (Paris), 175*(7-8):475-480. https://doi:10.1016/j.neurol.2019.07.005.

Tedder, D. G., Ashley, R., Tyler, K. L., & Levin, M. J. (1994). Herpes simplex virus infection as a cause of benign recurrent lymphocytic meningitis. *Ann Intern Med, 121*(5), 334-8. https://doi.org/10.7326/0003-4819-121-5-199409010-00004.

Thwaites, G., Fisher, M., Hemingway, C., Scott, G., Solomon, T., & Innes, J. (2009). British Infection Society guidelines for the diagnosis and treatment of tuberculosis of the central nervous system in adults and children. *J Infect, 59*, 167–187. https://doi.org/10.1016/j.jinf.2009.06.011.

Tyler, K. L. (2004). Herpes simplex virus infections of the central nervous system: encephalitis and meningitis, including *Mollaret's. Herpes, 11(*Suppl 2):57A-64A.

Verstrepen, W. A., Kuhn, S., Kockx, M. M., Van De Vyvere, M. E., & Mertens, A. H. (2001). Rapid detection of enterovirus RNA in cerebrospinal fluid specimens with a novel single-tube real-time reverse transcription-PCR assay. *J Clin Microbiol, 39*(11), 4093-6. https://doi:10.1128/JCM.39.11.4093-4096.2001.

Vinas, F. C., & Rengachary, S. (2001). Diagnosis and management of neurosarcoidosis. *J Clin Neurosci, 8*(6), 505-13. https://doi.org/10.1054/jocn.2000.0950.

Waghdhare, S., Kalantri, A., Joshi, R., & Kalantri, S. (2010). Accuracy of physical signs for detecting meningitis: a hospital-based diagnostic accuracy study. *Clin Neurol Neurosurg, 112*(9), 752-7. https://doi.org/10.1016/j.clineuro.2010.06.003.

Weiss, R. A. (1993). How does HIV cause AIDS? *Science, 260*(5112), 1273-9. https://doi.org/10.1126/science.8493571.

Zunt, J. R. (2002). Central nervous system infection during immunosuppression. *Neurol Clin, 20*(1), 1-22. https://doi.org/10.1016/s0733-8619(03)00070-7.

Chapter 5

Cerebrospinal Fluid Shunt Infections

Mehmet O. Bıyık*, MD
and Mehmet Aktoklu, MD
Departmant of Neurosurgery, Karadeniz Technical University, Trabzon, Turkiye

Abstract

For various reasons, 5-10% of shunt infections can be seen after the shunt set. It is more common, especially in the pediatric group. The current situation may result in serious morbidity and mortality in the patient. Apart from the difficulties that shunt infections bring to the patient, they also create serious costs such as prolonged hospitalization, long-term use of antibiotics, repeat surgical interventions, the need for palliative care that may occur after morbidity, psychosocial support, etc. Research on preventive and therapeutic methods, techniques, and shunt systems is still ongoing. It was aimed to present the subject together with the current articles in the literature related to shunt infections.

Keywords: hydrocephalus, ventriculoperitoneal shunt, shunt infections, infection management

Introduction

Hydrocephalus is a condition in which the dynamics of production, absorption, and circulation of the cerebrospinal fluid (CSF) are impaired due to various reasons or the enlargement of the ventricles as a result of developmental delay

* Corresponding Author's Email: mehmetorbaybyk@yahoo.com.

In: Central Nervous System Infections
Editor: Mustafa Usanmaz
ISBN: 979-8-89113-660-1

or atrophy of the brain tissue. Its prevalence is 88/100,000 in the pediatric population, 11/100,000 in adults, 175/100,000 in the elderly, and >400/100,000 in those over 80 years of age (Isaacs et al., 2018). Although increased intracranial pressure varies depending on the development time and speed, it can lead to various neurological symptoms ranging from headache to an increase in head circumference and death. Various shunt systems, such as ventriculoperitoneal (VP), ventriculoatrial (VA), ventriculopleural, and ventriculocysternal (Torkildsen) are used to transfer CSF to another body cavity in order to prevent brain damage, neurological deterioration, and provide recovery. Most commonly, a ventriculoperitoneal shunt (VPS) is used (Muram et al., 2022; Khan et al., 2022). Although VPS is more common in the first year, complications such as hematoma around the catheter, excessive drainage, mechanical dysfunction, pseudocyst, and most often misplacement and infections may develop (Ahmadvand et al., 2020; Yang et al., 2020; Colombo et al., 2022; Topçu et al., 2015). The frequency of shunt infection varies between 0.17-33%, but the general average and accepted range is 5-10%, and it is usually seen in the first six months after surgery and especially in newborns (Elsayed Saleh & Abou El Fetoh, 2023; Ayhan, 2022; Salek et al., 2022; Gülşen et al., 2015). Shunt infection is a complication that can cause serious mortality and morbidity in which leptomeningeal surfaces, CSF, and brain parenchyma are affected. At the same time, the development of intraventricular empyema not only causes severe damage to the brain parenchyma, but also creates a complex multilocular ventricle. Even if treated, they can cause neurological deficits and mental retardation (Topçu et al., 2015; Park, 2022). Even though the symptoms can vary, meningeal irritation is frequently accompanied by headache, drowsiness, vomiting, nausea, and neck stiffness. Fever, unsteady walking, convulsions, vision loss, stomach pain, erythema or edema along the shunt, and pseudocysts are further concerns (Yang et al., 2020). There are many risk elements such as the patient's age, additional diseases, weight, subcutaneous adipose tissue thickness, hydrocephalus type, surgical time, surgeon's experience, population of the operating room, and postoperative care (Salek et al., 2022; Yang et al., 2020). Typically, shunt infections occur a few days after surgery, on average in the first month. Standardized shunt infection prevention protocols have been shown to be a successful method to lower the frequency of shunt infections (Kestle et al., 2011; Muram et al., 2022).

Epidemiology – Incidence

VPS infections range between 0.17-33% (Gülşen et al., 2015). Kulkami detected shunt infections in 31 (10.4%) of 299 patients in a tertiary pediatric hospital between 1996 and 1999 (Kulkarni et al., 2001). In 333 VP shunt series retrospective cohort analysis at Korea Seoul National University Children's Hospital between January 2005 and February 2011, infection was observed in 35 shunts (10.5%) by Lee et al., and they observed that infection took place an average of 1 month (6 days to 8 months) after surgery (Lee et al., 2012). Between January 1, 2001, and December 31, 2005, a retrospective cohort analysis was carried out by Simon et al., in a series of 7071 cases aged 0-18 years with shunt registered in the Pediatric Health Information System (PHIS) by 41 pediatric hospitals, 825 (11.7%) detected shunt infection (Simon et al., 2009). Reddy et al. found infection in 107 of the 1015 patients who received ventriculoperitoneal shunt surgery between 1961 and 2010 in the retrospective analysis. 67 patients (6.6%) experienced a single infection attack, while 40 patients (3.9%) experienced numerous infections episodes. 7.2% of people worldwide were infected. The overall infection rate was 5.1% for adults and 9.5% for pediatric patients (Reddy et al., 2012). In the Hydrocephalus Clinical Research Network (HCRN) in 4 centers, a protocol was developed in order to lower the possibility of VPS infection, 1571 procedures were performed with 21 surgeons, and they created a network that they followed for a minimum of 6 months. According to that network has been reported that, the infection rate reduced from 8.8% before the protocol to 5.7% after the protocol was applied (Kestle et al., 2011).

Pathogenesis

The majority of shunt infections are brought on by the patient's skin, nose, and ears becoming contaminated with commensal organisms at the time of implantation, and some studies have even shown that 31% of skin swabs taken immediately after skin preparation with iodine scrub are positive, and again, it has shown that 25% of the swabs taken from surgical wounds are contaminated after the incision. Therefore, Coagulase negative staphylococci, S. aureus, and P. acnes are the organisms that most commonly cause infection (Walcott et al., 2012; Zervos & Walters, 2019; McGirt et al., 2003).

Risk Factors

Many variables have been studied that raise the possibility of shunt infection. For example, when Choudhury et al. evaluated 33 patients (20 under 1 year old) who underwent shunt surgery between 2015 and 2018, shunt infection was more typical in women, infants, and those with low socioeconomic status. In the same study, although it was not statistically significant between obstructive HS and contagious HS, slightly more infections were found in obstructive hydrocephalus. Infection was observed more frequently in cases whose operative time lasted longer than 1 hour (19 vs. 14) (15.2% vs. 9.1%). The most common type of shunt system was Codman (25 vs. 8), but in this group, shunt infection was only marginally more prevalent (5 vs. 3) and was not statistically significant. In the same study, when emergency and routine surgeries were evaluated, shunt infection (18.2% vs. 6.1%) was found to be higher in those who underwent emergency surgery (Salek et al., 2022). According to the research Matthew J. McGirt et al. conducted, infection developed in 92 shunts (11%) on average 19 days after the operation, according to 820 ventriculoperitoeal (VP) shunt placement data in 442 pediatric patients they examined. They observed the placement of a VP shunt in premature newborns, an approximately 5-fold increase in the risk of shunt infection, and with each passing year of patient age, the risk of shunt infection increases by 4%. It was determined that the use of an intraoperative neuroendoscope for shunt placement raised the risk of shunt infection 1.6 times. It has been determined that the risk of shunt insertion after a previous shunt infection increases approximately four times. They evaluated preterm delivery, previous shunt infection, and intraoperative neuroendoscope use as independent risk factors for shunt infection (McGirt et al., 2003). In the study of Amir Erps and his friends in 1570 patients; Shunt revision (2 or more), prolonged operation time, CSF leakage after surgery, and children younger than 5 years old were also found to be at high risk of infection. It was observed that the infection was lower in those with shunts due to neoplastic reasons, but the neoplastic group was older than the non-neoplastic ones. There were no appreciable differences between taking the first case or the last case. There was no significant difference between the use of an antibiotic-impregnated shunt and the normal shunt (Erps et al., 2018). In Yun-Na Yang et al. retrospective study on 502 patients; When tumors/cysts, cerebral hemorrhage, post-traumatic, postcraniotomy, aqueduct stenosis, spinal dysraphism, meningitis and congenital causes of hydrocephalus were evaluated, there was no statistically significant difference in the rate of intracranial infection between patients with different types of hydrocephalus. There were no appreciable differences between men and women. The average age of the patients was 57.1 ± 10.1. Among them, patients over 60 years of age had a higher rate of intracranial infection than patients under 60, and this difference was statistically significant. Age, skin infection, diabetes, and bedridden were associated with intracranial infection. The incidence of cerebral infection did not differ significantly among the various forms of hydrocephalus. It has been observed that changes in routine surgery, such as preserving the periosteum, closing the concealed puncture hole, a small curved scalp incision, and the use of preventive antibiotics, can reduce the risk of intracranial infection (Yang et al., 2020). Premature newborns with an immature immune system have been reported to be the group most at risk for shunt infections. A study found that a gestational age of <40 weeks was associated with a 2.05 greater probability of shunt failure due to infection, while another study found a 5-fold increased risk of shunt infection with shunt placement in a premature newborn. Although late shunt infections have also been reported, the majority of shunt infections occur within the first few weeks to several months after VPS insertion. Although contamination during shunt placement is typically the cause of early shunt infections, peritonitis, abdominal pseudocysts, hematogenous inoculations, and bowel perforations have also been observed as causes of late infections (Paff et al., 2018). In addition, it has been demonstrated that premature cases of posthemorrhagic hydrocephalus (PHH) have a higher risk of shunt infection, and the increase in CSF protein level and excess red blood cells have been reported to be the main reason for shunt failure and infection in these cases (Köksal & Öktem, 2010). The use of broad-spectrum antibiotics, corticosteroids, hyperalimentation, and immunosuppression increases the risk of fungal infection. Montero et al. reported that a 6-17% rate of fungal shunt infections was seen in their series (Montero et al., 2000).

To summarize risk factors; there is an increase in certain situations:

- Age (<5y and >60y), Female gender, Prematurity (<40h), Weight, Subcutaneous adipose tissue thickness, Socioeconomic status, Co-morbidities (diabetes, skin infections, bedridden condition, immunodeficiency), post-hemorrhagic hydrocephalus (especially in premature infants)
- Emergency surgery, Peritonitis, Intestine perforation, Abdominal pseudocyst

- Use of neuroendoscope, Number of people in the operating room, Surgeon's experience (<5 years), Surgery time (>1 hour)
- Postoperative care, CSF leakage after surgery, Re-shunt after shunt infection, Number of shunt revisions (>2), Corticosteroid use, Hyperalimentation

There is a decrease in certain conditions:

- Small, curved incision, Stitching the puncture hole buried, Keeping the periosteum intact, Wearing double gloves, Complying with and following up-to-date shunt protocols.

Causative Etiological Agents

The most frequently isolated organisms from infected shunts are Staphylococcus Epidermidis, Staphylococcus Aureus, and Gram-negative rods, in that order. Staphylococcus epidermidis and Staphylococcus Aureus are prevalent skin flora, and contamination of the skin usually causes infection during shunt insertion (Zervos & Walters, 2019; McGirt et al., 2003; Paff et al., 2018). Therefore, infections due to these organisms usually occur comparatively early after shunt placement. Staphylococcus aureus and Coagulase-negative Staphylococcus species, various Gram-negative rods, Proprionibacterum species, and Enterococcus faecalis are important factors of shunt infection (Topçu et al., 2015; McGirt et al., 2003). Microorganisms isolated less frequently are Gram negatives such as Escherichia coli, Klebsiella pneumonia, Proteus, and Pseudomonas, and Enterococcus. Fungal shunt infections are rarely encountered (Çağan et al., 2015; Fulkerson et al., 2011).

Clinical Findings

Patients who exhibit signs of shunt failure should always be suspected of being infected since shunt infection is a major complication with a high risk of serious morbidity and mortality. Patients frequently present with signs of a malfunctioning shunt as well as infection symptoms that are fever, but this is not always the case. Nausea, vomiting, headache, and fever may occur in patients with shunt failure for any reason, but fever is more common in patients with shunt infections (Paff et al., 2018). The most common findings are fever, local inflammation, restlessness (in the pediatric group), abdominal pain, seizure, and neurological changes (Paff et al., 2018; Lee et al., 2012). Above 38°C, fever, neck stiffness, decreased Glasgow Coma Scale, headache, nausea, signs of local infection, local pain, erythema, swelling, and/or purulent wound discharge may be observed (Paff et al., 2018; Lee et al., 2012; Conen et al., 2008). Fever and progressive unconsciousness are the most typical clinical characteristics in the adult patient group, while impaired consciousness and abdominal symptoms and findings are the most typical clinical characteristics in the pediatric patient group (Wang et al., 2004; Yakut et al., 2018).

Evaluation according to the ventriculitis and meningitis guide of 2017 Infectious Diseases Society of America's Clinical Practice (IDAH) (Tunkel et al., 2017):

- New headache, nausea, drowsiness, and/or change in mental state suggest cerebrospinal fluid (CSF) shunt infection.
- Redness and tenderness on the subcutaneous shunt tube suggest CSF shunt infection.
- Fever in the absence of another obvious source of infection may suggest CSF shunt infection.
- In the absence of another clear etiology, signs and symptoms of peritonitis or abdominal tenderness in patients with ventriculoperitoneal shunts are indicative of CSF shunt infection.
- In the absence of a different obvious cause in patients with ventriculopleural shunt, pleuritis symptoms, and signs are indicative of CSF shunt infection.
- Evidence of a CSF shunt infection is the presence of bacteremia in a patient with a ventriculoatrial shunt when there is no other clear source of bacteremia.
- A ventriculoatrial shunt patient's demonstration of glomerulonephritis raises the possibility of CSF shunt infection.
- Patients who have external ventricular drainage, a new or worsening mental status change is suggestive of infection.
- Patients with external ventricular drainage, new fever, and an increase in CSF leukocyte count may indicate infection.

Diagnostic Methods

The first step in diagnosis begins with a careful history and analysis of clinical findings and CSF and peripheral blood. Detailed neurological and systemic examination should be performed, and then the shunt trace should be checked for fluctuation and sensitivity by inspection and palpation.

Imaging

With direct radiographs, shunt continuity, the location of the ventricular tip, and whether it is short due to the growth of shunts inserted in the abdomen, especially in childhood, are evaluated throughout the abdomen. With uncontrasted brain CT and abdominal CT, the relationship between the shunt ventricul and intra-abdominal location, hemorrhages, pseudocysts, and intra-abdominal organs are evaluated. Ependymal staining with the contrast-enhanced abdomen and brain CT evaluates ventriculitis, cystic formations, and abscesses. Pseudocysts are evaluated with abdominal USG.

Diagnostic CSF Analysis

In cases of suspected shunt infection, a CSF sample should be taken by puncture from the shunt reservoir, through the catheter, or from the valve, CSF biochemistry, CSF culture, and Gram staining of CSF should be studied. If the shunt is removed, the shunt components (cranial tip, peritoneal tip, valve, etc.) should also be sent to culture (Elsayed Saleh & Abou El Fetoh, 2023; Çağan et al., 2015; Tunkel et al., 2017). It should not be forgotten that the shunt may also be contaminated during puncture and the mechanism may be disrupted. The area to be punctured is shaved, then cleaned with iodinated solution, then the necessary samples are taken by entering with a 25 gauge or finer needle (if possible, with a blunt tip). Positive CSF cultures, >10/mm3 leukocytes in CSF (this limit is 32/mm3 in newborns), protein level >45mg/dl (over 90 mg/dl in newborns) and decreased glucose ratios with accompanying fever, shunt dysfunction, neurological deterioration and is diagnosed by clinical findings such as abdominal symptoms. However, it should be kept in mind that pleocytosis can occur without infection, and infection can occur at normal protein and glucose levels (Paff et al., 2018; Çağan et al., 2015; Tunkel et al., 2017). A negative CSF Gram stain does not rule out the existence of infection, principally in individuals who have already undergone antibiotic medication, it should not be overlooked (Tunkel et al., 2017). It is advised to keep CSF cultures for at least ten days in patients with suspected CSF shunts or drainages if initial CSF cultures are negative to look for organisms such as Propionibacterium acnes (Tunkel et al., 2017). Blood cultures are recommended for those with ventriculoatrial shunts (Tunkel et al., 2017).

Treatment

After the shunt infection is diagnosed, systemic antimicrobial therapy should be started, and the shunt should be surgically removed. Since the causative agent is colonized on the catheter, the shunt and all of its elements must be removed from the CSF circulation for the treatment to be curative. Initially, external ventricular drainage (EVD) or a reservoir is attached and bactericidal effect drugs with good passage into CSF are started until the culture and antibiogram are concluded. It is recommended to include affected Gram-positive microorganisms because they are frequently seen (Elsayed Saleh & Abou El Fetoh, 2023; Zervos & Walters, 2019; Paff et al., 2018; Tunkel et al., 2017; Konrad et al., 2022; Shurtleff et al., 1974; Whitehead, W & Kestle, 2001; Schreffler et al., 2002). Empirical treatment for shunt infection should be based on pathogens commonly isolated in patients with shunt infection in that application setting and their susceptibility; however, a third-generation cephalosporin with a Gram-positive coating is recommended for general intravenous administration. Meropenem and/or higher antibiotics should be reserved for empirical treatment given for situations considered to be of high probability of hospital-acquired infections caused by broad-spectrum beta-lactamase-producing gram-negative bacilli (ESBL-GNB and Acinetobacter baumannii) (Udayakumaran et al., 2021).

Treatment according to the ventriculitis and meningitis guide of 2017 Infectious Diseases Society of America's Clinical Practice (IDAH) (Tunkel et al., 2017):

- -Nafcillin or oxacillin is recommended for the treatment of infection by Methicillin-susceptible Coagulase-negative staphylococci and S. aureus, and vancomycin as first-line therapy for infection by Methicillin-resistant Coagulase-negative staphylococci and S. aureus.
- Rifampin may be used in conjunction with other antimicrobial drugs if the staphylococcal isolate is rifampin-susceptible; this is especially advised as part of combination therapy in all patients with shunts.

- S. aureus infections should be treated for ten to 14 days whether they have systemic symptoms or not, CSF pleocytosis, or CSF glucose levels below 45 mg/dL.
- Patients receiving adequate antibiotic medication and having several positive CSF cultures should continue the treatment ten to 14 days after the most recent positive culture.
- Ten days after CSF cultures are negative, a new shunt should be implanted in patients with S. aureus infections.
- For the treatment of infections brought on by Propionibacterium acnes, penicillin G is advised. Treatment should last ten days for infections with little no CSF pleocytosis, normal CSF glucose, and few clinical signs or systemic characteristics.
- Patients without CSF abnormalities and whose CSF cultures are negative for 48 hours after VPS externalization should have a new shunt reimplanted in infections caused by coagulase-negative staphylococci and Propionibacterium acnes on the third day after removal; however, in patients with CSF abnormalities and negative repeated CSF cultures, a new shunt should be implanted after 7 days of antimicrobial therapy; and if repeat cultures are positive, antimicrobial
- For the treatment of infection by Gram-negative bacilli, third-generation cephalosporins with excellent CNS penetration are advised. For the cure of infections caused by Gram-negative bacilli that are sensitive, ceftriaxone or cefotaxime should be used, while meropenem should be used for infections caused by Gram-negative bacilli that produce extended-spectrum beta-lactamases.
- Clinical symptoms, CSF pleocytosis, CSF glucose 45mg/dL, or systemic Gram-negative bacilli infections, whether they have characteristics or not, should be treated for 10 to 14 days. Some doctors even advise treating these infections for 21 days. Treatment should be continued in patients receiving effective antibiotic therapy despite repeated positive CSF cultures for 10 to 14 days following the most recent positive culture.
- Ten days after CSF cultures are negative, a new shunt should be implanted in patients with infections brought on by Gram-negative bacilli.
- Cefepime, ceftazidime, or meropenem are suggested treatments for infections caused by Pseudomonas species.

- For the treatment of infections brought on by Acinetobacter species, meropenem is advised.

Conclusion

Various shunt systems such as ventriculoperitoneal (VP), ventriculoatrial (VA), ventriculopleural, and ventriculocysternal (Torkildsen) are used to transfer CSF to another body cavity in order to prevent brain damage, neurological deterioration, and provide recovery. Most commonly, a ventriculoperitoneal shunt (VPS) is used (Muram et al., 2022; Khan et al., 2022). The frequency of shunt infection varies between 0.17-33%, but the general average and accepted range is 5-10%, and it is usually seen in the first six months after surgery and especially in newborns (Elsayed Saleh & Abou El Fetoh, 2023; Ayhan, 2022; Salek et al., 2022; Gülşen et al., 2015). Most shunt infections result from contamination with commensal organisms in the patient's skin, nose, and ears at the time of implantation, therefore, Coagulase negative staphylococci, S. aureus, and P. acnes are the organisms that most commonly cause infection (Zervos & Walters, 2019; McGirt et al., 2003). Patients often present with shunt failure symptoms as well as infection symptoms, e.g., fever. Fever and progressive unconsciousness are the most typical clinical characteristics in the adult patient group, while impaired consciousness and abdominal symptoms and findings are the most typical clinical characteristics in the pediatric patient group (Wang et al., 2004; Yakut et al., 2018). In cases of suspected shunt infection, a CSF sample should be taken by puncture from the shunt reservoir, through the catheter, or from the valve, CSF biochemistry, CSF culture, and Gram staining of CSF should be studied. If the shunt is removed, shunt components (cranial tip, peritoneal tip, valve, etc.) should also be sent to culture (Topçu et al., 2015; Çağan et al., 2015; Tunkel et al., 2017). It should not be forgotten that the shunt may also be contaminated during puncture and the mechanism may be disrupted. Positive CSF cultures, >10/mm3 leukocytes in CSF (this limit is 32/mm3 in newborns), protein level >45mg/dl (over 90 mg/dl in newborns), and decreased glucose ratios with accompanying fever, shunt dysfunction, neurological deterioration and it is diagnosed by clinical findings such as abdominal symptoms. However, it should be kept in mind that pleocytosis can occur without infection, and infection can occur at normal protein and glucose levels (Paff et al., 2018, Çağan et al., 2015; Tunkel et al., 2017). A negative

CSF Gram stain does not rule out the existence of infection, especially in individuals who have already undergone antibiotic medication, it should not be missed (Tunkel et al., 2017). After the shunt infection is diagnosed, systemic antimicrobial therapy should be started, and the shunt should be surgically removed. Since the causative agent is colonized on the catheter, the shunt and all of its elements must be removed from the CSF circulation for the treatment to be curative. Initially, external ventricular drainage (EVD) or a reservoir is attached and bactericidal effect drugs with good passage into the CSF are started until the culture and antibiogram are concluded. It is recommended to include affected Gram-positive microorganisms because they are frequently seen (Elsayed Saleh & Abou El Fetoh, 2023; Zervos & Walters, 2019; Paff et al., 2018; Tunkel et al., 2017; Konrad et al., 2022; Shurtleff et al., 1974; Whitehead, W & Kestle, 2001; Schreffler et al., 2002).

Since the most effective method is prevention, the necessary prophylaxis and sterility rules should be followed, the operation should be performed as soon as possible under elective conditions by experienced surgeons with few people, and regular attention should be paid to postoperative care. The necessary training should be given to the patients and their relatives for the post-hospital period.

References

Ahmadvand, S., Dayyani, M., Etemadrezaie, H., Ghorbanpour, A., Zarei, R., Shahriyari, A., Emadzadeh, M., Ganjeifar, B., & Zabihyan, S. (2020). Rate and risk factors of early ventriculoperitoneal shunt revision: a five-year retrospective analysis of a referral center. *World Neurosurgery*, *134*, e505-e511. https://doi.org/10.1016/j.wneu.2019.10.108.

Ayhan, L. (2022). *Ventriküloperitoneal şant cerrahisi uygulanan pediatrik hidrosefali olgularının retrospektif değerlendirilmesi [Retrospective evaluation of pediatric hydrocephalus cases who underwent ventriculoperitoneal shunt surgery]* (Medical Specialist Thesis). Meram Medicine Faculty, Necmettin Erbakan University, Konya, Turkiye.

Colombo, E. V., Bongetta, D., Cofano, F., Versace, A., Garbossa, D., Bertuccio, A., Armocida, D., d'Auria, P., Farina, L. M., Assietti, R., & Tartara, F. (2022). Ventricular Peritoneal Shunting Using Modified Keen's Point Approach: Technical Report and Cases Series. *Surgeries*, *3*(4), 314-322. https://doi.org/10.3390/surgeries3040034.

Conen, A., Walti, L. N., Merlo, A., Fluckiger, U., Battegay, M., & Trampuz, A. (2008). Characteristics and treatment outcome of cerebrospinal fluid shunt-associated infections in adults: a retrospective analysis over an 11-year period. *Clinical infectious diseases*, *47*(1), 73-82. https://doi.org/10.1086/588298.

Çağan, E., Soysal, A., Şeker, A., & Şeker, M. (2015). Ventriculoperitoneal shunt infection and treatment in children. *Cukurova Medical Journal*, *40*(1), 72-79. https://doi.org/10.17826/cutf.09848.

Elsayed Saleh, A., & Abou El Fetoh, I. (2023). Outcome of Antibiotic-Impregnated Shunt (AIS) Catheters for Management of Hydrocephalus: A Retro-Prospective Study versus Non-AIS Catheters. *Benha Medical Journal*, *40*(Special issue (Surgery)), 1-14. https://doi.org/10.21608/bmfj.2022.265457.

Erps, A., Roth, J., Constantini, S., Lerner-Geva, L., & Grisaru-Soen, G. (2018). Risk factors and epidemiology of pediatric ventriculoperitoneal shunt infection. *Pediatrics International*, *60*(12), 1056-1061. https://doi.org/10.1086/368191.

Fulkerson, D. H., Sivaganesan, A., Hill, J. D., Edwards, J. R., Shoja, M. M., Boaz, J. C., & Jea, A. (2011). Progression of cerebrospinal fluid cell count and differential over a treatment course of shunt infection. *Journal of Neurosurgery: Pediatrics*, *8*(6), 613-619. https://doi.org/10.3171/2011.8.PEDS11236.

Gülşen, İ., Ak, H., Aycan, A., Atalay, T., Sösuncu, E., Akyol, M. E., Kuyumcu, F. & Arslan, M. (2015). Pediatrik Şant Enfeksiyonları: 105 Olguluk Çift Merkezli Çalışma [Pediatric Shunt Infections: Two centered Study with 105 Cases]. *Bozok Tıp Dergisi*, 5(1), 13-17.

Isaacs, A. M., Riva-Cambrin, J., Yavin, D., Hockley, A., Pringsheim, T. M., Jette, N., Lethebe BC, Lowerison M, Dronyk J, & Hamilton, M. G. (2018). Age-specific global epidemiology of hydrocephalus: Systematic review, metanalysis and global birth surveillance. *PloS one*, *13*(10), e0204926. https://doi.org/10.1371/journal.pone.0210851.

Kestle, J. R., Riva-Cambrin, J., Wellons, J. C., Kulkarni, A. V., Whitehead, W. E., Walker, M. L., Oakes, W. J., Drake, J. M., Luerssen, T. G., Simon, T. D., & Holubkov, R. (2011). A standardized protocol to reduce cerebrospinal fluid shunt infection: the Hydrocephalus Clinical Research Network Quality Improvement Initiative. *Journal of Neurosurgery: Pediatrics*, *8*(1), 22-29. https://doi.org/10.3171/2011.4.PEDS10551.

Khan, Z., Sharafat, S., Nazir, R., & Younis, F. (2022). A Prospective Study on Ventriculoperitoneal Shunt Surgery Complications in Tertiary Care Hospital. *Journal of Pharmaceutical Negative Results*, 592-598. https://doi.org/10.47750/pnr.2022.13.S09.65.

Konrad, E., Robinson, J. L., & Hawkes, M. T. (2022). Cerebrospinal fluid shunt infections in children. *Archives of Disease in Childhood*. https://doi.org/10.1136/archdischild-2022-324559.

Köksal, V., & Öktem, S. (2010). Ventriculosubgaleal shunt procedure and its long-term outcomes in premature infants with post-hemorrhagic hydrocephalus. *Child's Nervous System*, *26*, 1505-1515. https://doi.org/10.1007/s00381-010-1118-x.

Kulkarni, A. V., Drake, J. M., & Lamberti-Pasculli, M. (2001). Cerebrospinal fluid shunt infection: a prospective study of risk factors. *Journal of neurosurgery*, *94*(2), 195-201. https://doi.org/10.3171/jns.2001.94.2.0195.

Lee, J. K., Seok, J. Y., Lee, J. H., Choi, E. H., Phi, J. H., Kim, S. K., Wang, K. C., & Lee, H. J. (2012). Incidence and risk factors of ventriculoperitoneal shunt infections in children: a study of 333 consecutive shunts in 6 years. *Journal of Korean medical science*, *27*(12), 1563-1568. https://doi.org/10.3346/jkms.2012.27.12.1563.

McGirt, M. J., Zaas, A., Fuchs, H. E., George, T. M., Kaye, K., & Sexton, D. J. (2003). Risk factors for pediatric ventriculoperitoneal shunt infection and predictors of infectious pathogens. *Clinical infectious diseases*, *36*(7), 858-862.

Montero, A., Romero, J., Vargas, J. A., Regueiro, C. A., Sanchez-Aloz, G., De Prados, F., De la Torre, A., & Aragon, G. (2000). Candida infection of cerebrospinal fluid shunt devices: report of two cases and review of the literature. *Acta neurochirurgica*, *142*, 67-74. https://doi.org/10.1007/s007010050009.

Muram, S., Isaacs, A. M., Sader, N., Holubkov, R., Fong, A., Conly, J., & Hamilton, M. G. (2022). A standardized infection prevention bundle for reduction of CSF shunt infections in adult ventriculoperitoneal shunt surgery performed without antibiotic-impregnated catheters. *Journal of Neurosurgery*, *1*(aop), 1-9. https://doi.org/10.3171/2022.5.JNS22430.

Muram, S., Isaacs, A. M., Sader, N., Holubkov, R., Fong, A., Conly, J., & Hamilton, M. G. (2022). A standardized infection prevention bundle for reduction of CSF shunt infections in adult ventriculoperitoneal shunt surgery performed without antibiotic-impregnated catheters. *Journal of Neurosurgery*, *132*(8), 494-502. https://doi.org/10.3171/2022.5.JNS22430.

Paff, M., Alexandru-Abrams, D., Muhonen, M., & Loudon, W. (2018). Ventriculoperitoneal shunt complications: a review. *Interdisciplinary Neurosurgery*, *13*, 66-70. https://doi.org/10.1016/j.inat.2018.04.004.

Park, Y. S. (2022). Treatment Strategies and Challenges to Avoid Cerebrospinal Fluid Shunting for Pediatric Hydrocephalus. *Neurologia medico-chirurgica*, *62*(9), 416-430. https://doi.org/10.2176/jns-nmc.2022-0100.

Reddy, G. K., Bollam, P., & Caldito, G. (2012). Ventriculoperitoneal shunt surgery and the risk of shunt infection in patients with hydrocephalus: long-term single institution experience. *World neurosurgery*, *78*(1-2), 155-163. https://doi.org/10.1016/j.wneu.2011.10.034.

Salek, M. A. A., Faisal, H., & Islam, M. A. (2022). Ventriculo-Peritoneal Shunt Infection: Three Years Experience in Combined Military Hospital, Dhaka. *Journal of Armed Forces Medical College, Bangladesh*, *18*(1), 16-18. https://doi.org/10.3329/jafmc.v18i1.61250.

Schreffler, R. T., Schreffler, A. J., & Wittler, R. R. (2002). Treatment of cerebrospinal fluid shunt infections: a decision analysis. *The Pediatric infectious disease journal*, *21*(7), 632-636.

Shurtleff, D. B., Foltz, E. L., Weeks, R. D., & Loeser, J. (1974). Therapy of Staphylococcus epidermidis: Infections associated with cerebrospinal fluid shunts. *Pediatrics*, *53*(1), 55-62. https://doi.org/10.1542/peds.53.1.55.

Simon, T. D., Hall, M., Riva-Cambrin, J., Albert, J. E., Jeffries, H. E., LaFleur, B., Dean, J. M., & Kestle, J. R. (2009). Infection rates following initial cerebrospinal fluid shunt placement across pediatric hospitals in the United States. *Journal of Neurosurgery: Pediatrics*, *4*(2), 156-165. https://doi.org/10.3171/2009.3.PEDS08215.

Topçu, A., Gedik Topçu, B., Korucu, M., Ünal, M. S., Turgut, S., & Çırak, B. (2015). Ratlarda Deneysel Epilepsi Modelinde İntrahipokampal ve İntravasküler Allojenik Kök Hücre Uygulamasının İktal Aktivite Üzerine Etkilerinin Araştırılması [Investigation of the Effects of Intrahippocampal and Intravascular Allogeneic Stem

Cell Application on Ictal Activity in Experimental Epilepsy Model in Rats.]. *29th Scientific Congress of Turkish Neurosurgical Society,* April 17 - 21, 2015, Antalya, Turkiye.

Tunkel, A. R., Hasbun, R., Bhimraj, A., Byers, K., Kaplan, S. L., Scheld, W. M., van de Beek, D., Bleck, T. P., Garton, H. J. L., & Zunt, J. R. (2017). 2017 Infectious Diseases Society of America's clinical practice guidelines for healthcare-associated ventriculitis and meningitis. *Clinical Infectious Diseases*, *64*(6), e34-e65. https://doi.org/10.1093/cid/ciw861.

Udayakumaran, S., Pillai, S., Dwarakanath, S., Bhattacharjee, S., Mehrotra, N., Raju, S., Gupta, D., Panigrahi, M., Venkataramana, N. K., Rajshekhar, V., & Sankhla, S. (2021). Indian Society of Pediatric Neurosurgery Consensus Guidelines on Preventing and Managing Shunt Infection: Version 2020-21. *Neurology India*, *69*(Supplement), S526–S555. https://doi.org/10.4103/0028-3886.332268.

Walcott, B. P., Redjal, N., & Coumans, J. V. C. (2012). Infection following operations on the central nervous system: deconstructing the myth of the sterile field. *Neurosurgical focus*, *33*(5), E8. https://doi.org/10.3171/2012.8.FOCUS12245.

Wang, K. W., Chang, W. N., Shih, T. Y., Huang, C. R., Tsai, N. W., Chang, C. S., Chuang, Y. C., Liliang, P. C., Su, T. M., Rau, C. S., Tsai, Y. D., Cheng, B. C., Hung, P. L., & Lu, C. H. (2004). Infection of cerebrospinal fluid shunts: causative pathogens, clinical features, and outcomes. *Japanese journal of infectious diseases*, *57*(2), 44-48. https://pubmed.ncbi.nlm.nih.gov/15118207/.

Whitehead, W. E., & Kestle, J. R. (2001). The treatment of cerebrospinal fluid shunt infections. *Pediatric neurosurgery*, *35*(4), 205-210. https://doi.org/10.1159/000050422.

Yakut, N., Soysal, A., Kepenekli Kadayifci, E., Dalgic, N., Yılmaz Ciftdogan, D., Karaaslan, A., Akkoc, G., Ocal Demir, S., Cagan, E., Celikboya, E., Kanik, A., Dagcinar, A., Yilmaz, A., Ozer, F., Camlar, M., Turel, O., & Bakir, M. (2018). Ventriculoperitoneal shunt infections and re-infections in children: a multicentre retrospective study. *British journal of neurosurgery*, *32*(2), 196-200. https://doi.org/10.1080/02688697.2018.1467373.

Yang, Y. N., Zhang, J., Gu, Z., & Song, Y. L. (2020). The risk of intracranial infection in adults with hydrocephalus after ventriculoperitoneal shunt surgery: a retrospective study. *International Wound Journal*, *17*(3), 722-728. https://doi.org/10.1111/iwj.13331.

Yang, Y. N., Zhang, J., Gu, Z., & Song, Y. L. (2020). The risk of intracranial infection in adults with hydrocephalus after ventriculoperitoneal shunt surgery: a retrospective study. *International Wound Journal*, *17*(3), 722-728. https://doi.org/10.1111/iwj.13331.

Zervos, T., & Walters, B. C. (2019). Diagnosis of Ventricular Shunt Infection in Children: A Systematic Review. *World neurosurgery*, *129*, 34–44. https://doi.org/10.1016/j.wneu.2019.05.057.

Chapter 6

Tuberculosis Meningitis

Elif Aydın*, **PhD**
Department of Medical Services and Techniques, Kutahya Health Sciences University, Tavşanlı Health Services Vocational School, Kütahya, Turkiye

Abstract

Tuberculous meningitis is the most severe and fatal form of extrapulmonary tuberculosis. Despite all advances in medicine, it is still a very difficult disease to diagnose. It begins with the development of tuberculosis foci in the brain, spinal cord, or meninges. Worldwide, about 1% of all tuberculosis cases and 5% of all extrapulmonary cases show central nervous system involvement, and it is more common in children and those with HIV infection. TB meningitis in adults often presents as a subacute/chronic febrile illness. Clinically, classic symptoms of meningitis such as fever, headache, nuchal rigidity, focal neurological findings, behavioral changes, and confusion are observed. Delays in diagnosis are associated with increased mortality and morbidity.

Keywords: tuberculous meningitis, mycobacterium tuberculosis, tuberculosis, extracardiac tuberculosis

Introduction

Central nervous system involvement is considered the most serious form of tuberculosis due to its high morbidity and mortality. In tuberculosis of the

---

* Corresponding Author's Email: elifkn@hotmail.com.

In: Central Nervous System Infections
Editor: Mustafa Usanmaz
ISBN: 979-8-89113-660-1

central nervous system, different clinical forms such as meningitis, focal cerebritis, intracranial tuberculoma, tubercular abscess, tubercular vasculopathy, infarction in the basal ganglia, and hydrocephalus may develop. Tuberculosis is less common in the spinal cord where arachnoiditis and intramedullary tuberculoma are seen. 95% of cases present as meningitis, 5% as tuberculoma, and less than 1% as abscess. The disease is most common in children aged 6 months to 4 years (Gupta and Kumar, 2011).

Meningitis, one of the central nervous system infections, is an acute or chronic inflammatory disease caused by microorganisms that damage brain membranes and tissues, characterized by cellular and biochemical changes in cerebrospinal fluid (CSF) and neurological findings in the clinic (Ellard et al., 1987). Inflammation of the pia and arachnoid membrane surrounding the brain and spinal cord is defined as meningitis. Significant changes are observed in the etiologic distribution depending on age, genetic structure, geographical differences, season, socioeconomic conditions, and local endemic factors (Ellard et al., 1987). Many agents including bacteria, viruses, fungi, protozoa, and some parasites can cause diseases in the CNS. The clinical course may be acute, subacute, or chronic depending on the type of infection. Acute purulent meningitis is usually bacterial, while acute aseptic meningitis is usually viral. Tuberculous meningitis is the leading cause of chronic meningitis. Treatment approaches rapidly reduce the mortality of bacterial meningitis, while viral meningitis has a milder course. However, it is known that the mortality or sequelae rate is high in tuberculous meningitis (Lewinsohn et al., 2017).

Tuberculosis is one of the oldest known diseases that continues to be an important public health problem in the world. It is estimated that 1.7 billion people, 1/3 of the world's population, are infected with tuberculosis bacilli, and 100-200 million people are added to this pool every year. Every year, 8 million people are infected with tuberculosis, 2 million people die from the disease, and 98% of these deaths occur in developing countries (WHO, 2019).

Tuberculous meningitis is an important form of tuberculosis with high morbidity and mortality and is observed in 5-10% of patients with tuberculosis and is the most severe clinical form of the disease. The clinical manifestations of tuberculous meningitis are highly variable and vary between populations (Ellard et al., 1987). Because of the rapid and devastating course of the disease, the diagnosis should be made early/quickly, and treatment should be started without delay. Laboratory examination of CSF may not always be helpful (Sheller and Des Prez, 1986). Therefore, the diagnosis of tuberculous meningitis is based on a combination of history, clinical, micrological, biochemical, and sometimes radiological investigations. The aim of early diagnosis of tuberculous meningitis is to start early treatment. Early treatment is also important in terms of preventing the development of neurologic complications. As a matter of fact, 100% recovery is achieved in patients who start treatment in the early period. Otherwise, the development of severe neurologic complications is inevitable in patients who are not treated for 3-8 weeks (Sheller and Des Prez, 1986).

Epidemiology

Tuberculous meningitis is the most severe clinical form of tuberculosis, and despite diagnostic and treatment modalities, the disease is associated with high mortality and sequelae rates. Tuberculous meningitis occurs in approximately 1% of patients with tuberculosis. The causative agent of tuberculous meningitis is generally Mycobacterium tuberculosis. Mycobacterium bovis and atypical mycobacteria may rarely be the causative agents of meningitis. Intracellular M. avium may be the causative agent of tuberculosis, especially in HIV-positive patients. The main characteristics of bacteria in the genus Mycobacterium are slow growth, acid resistance, and abundant lipids in the cell walls (Ellard et al., 1987). The incidence of tuberculous meningitis is parallel to the prevalence of tuberculosis in the community. This disease, which can be seen at any age, is most common in the first five years of childhood in underdeveloped or developing countries. In societies where the prevalence of TB is lower, most cases are seen in adults, with the highest incidence in the 25-45 age group. The disease usually develops as a complication of primary infection. The risk of developing meningitis in HIV-infected tuberculosis patients is approximately 5 times higher than in HIV-uninfected patients (Gray and Fedorko, 1992). This situation poses a particular threat to North America, Latin America, and Eastern Europe, as well as some Asian countries with large populations such as India, and geographies such as South-Saharan Africa. The etiologic distribution may vary with age, geographical differences, season, genetics, and susceptibility of the population to certain factors. There is genetic susceptibility to tuberculosis. It is believed that the black race is more susceptible due to a change in the NRAMP1 gene. (Tunkel et al., 2004).

Drug-resistant tuberculosis is one of the most worrying situations today. Although multidrug resistance rates of 8.6% in South Africa, 2.4% in India, and 2.4% in Vietnam have been found in various studies, it is not yet though to be a problem for tuberculous meningitis.

Several new vaccines against tuberculosis are promising for the fight against tuberculosis and, if successful, will reduce the incidence of tuberculous meningitis. Screening and treatment of individuals with latent tuberculosis can also help prevent tuberculosis (WHO, 2019).

Pathogenesis

Tuberculous meningitis may develop as an early or late complication of tuberculosis infection, or it may develop during the course of chronic tuberculosis infection or as an end-stage complication in untreated patients (Kasik, 1988). The disease begins with the inhalation of a small number of bacilli by inhalation of infected droplets scattered in the environment by coughing of a person with active pulmonary tuberculosis. Bacilli inhaled by the non-immune host reach extrapulmonary areas within the alveolar macrophages via the hematogenous route and initiate extrapulmonary tuberculosis. The bacilli spreading through the bloodstream can also settle in the central nervous system. Cellular immunity can kill the bacilli in this process. Necrotic caseous tissues surrounded by mononuclear cells, called tubercles, form in the lung and other areas and are an important stage in the development of tuberculosis infection. The disease develops when cellular immunity is deficient. After the suppression of cellular immunity, tuberculous meningitis may develop in patients either due to the hematogenous spread of the primary infection to the central nervous system or due to the opening of the subarachnoid space into the subarachnoid space due to the growth of existing tuberculoma foci and rupture of the caseous center of the bacteria multiplying in them (Roca, 2005; Donald et al., 2004). Microorganisms can also reach the CNS through bony structures such as the middle ear or vertebrae. A small proportion of cases may develop from foci in the ventricular wall or choroid plexus. Tuberculous meningitis occurs in two stages. First, bacilli reach the central nervous system through hematogenous routes and form small intracerebral tuberculosis lesions called 'Rich Foci'. These lesions may be under the piamater or on the subependymal surface, and it is not known exactly how long they can remain. After this stage, small tuberculosis lesions located on the brain surface or ependyma open into the subarachnoid space or ventricle and lead to the development of meningitis. The lesions may lead to the development of tuberculomas or abscesses, either in the brain parenchyma or in the spinal cortex. The defense mechanism is very important in the development of these stages. Although the pathogenesis process after spreading from the Rich focus has not been clearly elucidated, it is thought that new developments will be made in the treatment of the disease and thus in its prognosis (Dastur et al., 1995; Thwaites et al., 2005).

In tuberculous meningitis, the meninges are frequently involved together with brain tissue. A thick gelatinous exudate spreads into the subarachnoid space. This exudate may spread from the initial focus of infection to the basal cisternae and sylvian fissure. In time, the exudate spreads to the lateral ventricles and covers the choroid plexus there. The exudate contains polymorphous nuclear leukocytes, lymphocytes, erythrocytes, macrophages, and a fibrin network, and tubercle bacilli within this fibrin network. Small arteries, veins, and capillary structures in the exudate area are also affected by this exudate and inflammation develops (Roca, 2005). Cranial nerves are affected by the cerebrospinal fluid circulation disorder caused by exudate, and granuloma structures may turn into tuberculomas and abscesses. The severity of complications in cases of tuberculous meningitis is related to the severity of the inflammatory response in the head (Katti, 2004; Thwaites et al., 2005). An important characteristic of tuberculous meningitis is vasculitis; arteries and veins are involved, and aneurysms, thrombi, focal hemorrhagic infarcts, and obliterative vasculitis occur. Obstructive hydrocephalus may develop due to compression of the brainstem by the dense exudate in the meninges, and edema in the midbrain, or the obstructive effect of tuberculomas in the brainstem. In some cases, communicating hydrocephalus may develop with impaired CSF resorption. Involvement of the middle cerebral artery may cause hemiparesis. Vasculitis may lead to aneurysm, thrombosis, and focal hemorrhagic infarcts (cerebral ischemia). The most common vascular involvement in tuberculous meningitis is cerebral ischemia due to vascular occlusion (Chan et al., 2005).

Cominican hydrocephalus occurs with decreased absorption of cerebrospinal fluid from the basal cisterns. In addition, hydrocephalus may also develop as a result of the failure of the CSF to drain from the 4th ventricle, and obstruction of the aquaductus cerebrini with exudate, and atrophy of the white and gray matter develops in the absence of treatment (Katti, 2004; Thwaites et al., 2005).

Metabolic complications can also be seen in cases of tuberculous meningitis. Hyponatremia is the most common metabolic complication and can also be seen in inappropriate antidiuretic syndrome. However, despite normal levels of antidiuretic hormone (ADH) in many patients, persistent hyponatremia can be found in many patients. There is a strong correlation between plasma atrial natriuretic peptide and sodium concentrations in these patients. This picture seen in patients with tuberculous meningitis is often referred to as 'hyponatremic natriuretic syndrome' (Cotton et al., 1991).

Clinical Symptoms and Findings

The clinical spectrum of tuberculous meningitis is quite broad. It can range from chronic headache to altered consciousness, progressive meningitis, and coma. Initially, it is usually silent. Apathy, irritability, anorexia, fever, headache, and vomiting are common. Fever may be absent in up to 10% of patients.

Tuberculous meningitis has quite different clinical manifestations. Age and stage of the disease at the time of diagnosis are very important parameters in the clinical presentation of the patient. Furthermore, intense basilar exudation (cranial nerve involvement, hydrocephalus), vasculitis and vascular occlusion (focal neurological deficits), allergic reactions to tuberculoprotein (changes in CSF), cerebral edema (changes in consciousness, epileptic seizures, increased intracranial pressure) and the presence of tuberculomas acting as space-occupying lesions are factors responsible for the clinical picture. Clinical findings are associated with pathological changes and reflect changes in the CNS (Katti, 2004).

The clinical picture varies greatly from patient to patient. The misinterpretation of the prodromal symptoms of the disease has important consequences in terms of treatment and prognosis. Tuberculous meningitis has three clinical stages: prodromal, meningitic (meningeal irritation), and paralytic (cerebral involvement).

Prodromal Period

It may last for a few days to a few weeks. It may even last for a few months. Initial findings are non-specific complaints rather than disease-specific symptoms. They may include weakness, anorexia, mild fever, depression, confusion, personality changes, fatigue, muscle aches, and headache. In some adults, the prodrome period may present as slowly progressive dementia. During this period, personality changes, memory impairment, and loss of libido may be observed. There is no focal neurologic disorder at this stage. Generally, no diagnosis can be made at this stage (Mezochow et al., 2017).

Meningitic Period (Meningeal Irritation)

Shows a rapid onset. It is the period when neurological symptoms are more prominent. These are recognized as meningismus, severe headaches, vomiting, lethargy, confusion, vomiting, hypertonia, cranial nerve involvement and focal neurological involvement, and the addition of varying degrees of cranial nerve and spinal nerve signs and symptoms. The fundus is usually normal during this period. Some children may have encephalitis findings such as disorientation, abnormal movements, and speech disorders (Mezochow et al., 2017).

Paralytic Period (Cerebral Involvement)

Severe disturbances of consciousness, lethargy, confusion, stupor, and clinical findings leading to coma and frequent hemiparesis are observed. Findings indicating increased intracranial pressure become prominent and papillary edema appears. Disorders in CSF circulation and absorption lead to hydrocephalus. Hemiplegia or paraplegia is present. The patient is in a deceased or decorticated position. An increase in intracranial pressure is observed. In the terminal period, deep coma, decerebrate or decorticated posture, spasms and extensor rigidity, pupils dilate and flicker, pulse rate increases, respiration becomes irregular, and death follows this picture. Most patients without treatment die within 5-8 weeks after the onset of the disease (Kent et al., 1993).

The staging chart first developed by the 'British Medical Research Council' (BMC; BMR) in 1947 is still in use after modification. This classification is very useful in terms of prognosis and in organizing treatment for the patient (Joint Tuberculosis Committee of the British Thoracic Society, 1998).

- *Stage I:* Consciousness is clear, nonspecific symptoms are present, focal neurologic symptoms, hydrocephalus, and neurologic deficit are absent.
- *Stage II:* There is lethargy and confusion. There may be mild to severe focal signs and symptoms, such as cranial nerve palsy or cranial nerve hemiparesis.

- *Stage III:* Delirium, stupor, or marked paraplegia, coma, convulsions, multiple cranial nerve palsies, and/or intense.

Cranial nerve involvement occurs in 20-30% of patients with tuberculous meningitis and may be the first presenting symptom. The 6th, 3rd, 4th, and 7th cranial nerves are the most commonly affected pairs of cranial nerves, respectively. The 6th nerve is most commonly affected, and the 3rd and 4th nerves are less frequently affected. The 2nd cranial nerve can also be involved. Initially, the paralysis is unilateral, but later it becomes bilateral. The facial nerve is the least commonly involved nerve. Other cranial nerves are rarely affected; optic nerve involvement causes optic atrophy and blindness. Although generalized convulsions occur in children, focal seizures are more common in adults. In 10-15% of children, convulsive seizures are the presenting symptom or an early symptom (Katti, 2004; Mezochow et al., 2017).

In HIV-positive patients, the risk of developing tuberculous meningitis is higher in parallel with the risk of developing tuberculosis. In the presence of HIV positivity, the risk of developing tuberculous meningitis increases, and its progression is quite rapid. In the CSF of some HIV patients, the nucleic acid materials of tuberculosis bacilli can be detected without detecting cells. Although the clinical patterns are not different, the course of complications is aggravated, and the disease is serious. Basal meninges involvement and hydrocephalus are more common in this group (Berenguer et al., 1992).

Diagnostics

One of the most important challenges for tuberculous meningitis is the difficulty of diagnosis. The diagnosis should be made as early as possible without any change in consciousness or loss of consciousness in the early period. The most important clue in anamnesis is contact with a known tuberculosis case and previous tuberculosis. Chest radiographs show evidence of active or previous lung infection in almost half of the cases (van den Bos, 2004). In blood tests, patients may have low or normal leukocytes, erythrocyte sedimentation rate is usually high, mild anemia, hyponatremia, and hypokleremia due to inappropriate release of antidiuretic hormone (Gray and Fedorko, 1992). In HIV-infected patients, hilar lymphadenopathy on chest radiography is a more common finding than in other patients, while PPD positivity is a less common finding (Berenguer et al., 1992).

Tuberculin Test

A positive tuberculin test in children and adults is helpful in diagnosis. A negative result does not rule out the disease. In some cases, PPD may be positive during treatment. The skin test may be negative in patients with debility or malnutrition, those receiving corticosteroid therapy, immunosuppressed patients, and terminally ill patients.

Cerebrospinal Fluid (CSF) Examination

Three or four tubes are required for chemical or serological tests, hematologic, and microbiological investigations. If the intervention during CSF collection is traumatic, it is to prevent a falsely elevated white blood cell count and contamination of the skin flora and CSF culture sample. The CSF should be sent to the laboratory immediately after collection. It should never be left in the refrigerator except for molecular and virologic examinations (Bonsu and Harper, 2005).

Pressure discoloration, turbidity, erythrocyte and leukocyte cell count, protein and glucose concentration measurement, separation of cells, Gram staining, and bacterial culture are the tests performed in CSF examination. Findings should always be interpreted according to clinical, neurologic, and neuroradiological findings (Bonsu and Harper, 2005).

The first step in the examination of the CSF is to measure the opening pressure with an air-water manometer. The opening pressure of the CSF is between 50-195 mm H2O in healthy individuals. If the CSF pressure is very low and close to zero, the complete spinal block should be considered. In cases where it is too high, the risk of herniation should be considered and measures should be taken to reduce intracranial pressure.

The CSF is normally clear. The presence of more than 200 leukocytes per milliliter, more than 400 erythrocytes per mL, more than 10 5 cfu/mL of bacteria, and/or more than 150 mg/dL of protein causes the CSF to appear cloudy. Bloody if the erythrocyte count is more than 6000/mm3, turbid and xanthochromic if it is between 400-6000/mm3 (yellow or yellow-green coloration or pinkish appearance of centrifuged CSF supernatant) (Tülek and Fışkın, 2008).

Direct examination of CSF is important in differentiating subarachnoid hemorrhage from traumatic LP. While CSF is initially bloody after traumatic LP, its color lightens with time due to CSF flow. Coagulation in the tube is also in favor of traumatic LP. Traumatic LP makes the diagnosis difficult. Leukocyte and protein concentrations are affected by traumatic LP, but gram staining, culture, and glucose levels are not (Tülek and Tanyel, 2008).

Normally, there are no polymorphonuclear leukocytes (PMNL) in the CSF. If the cell count is ≥10/mm3, it is considered pathologic. In untreated bacterial meningitis, the white blood cell count in the CSF is usually between 1000-5000/mm3. This number varies between 100-10000 (Kanra, 1993).

Normally, the CSF protein is 15-45 mg/dL. The CSF protein increases in bacterial meningitis. This increase is due to disruption of the blood-brain barrier and inflammation. In cases where the protein is very high, the CSF spontaneously coagulates if left for a while. The normal glucose level in CSF examinations is 50-80 mg/dL, which is 60-70% of the blood glucose level. Since the CSF glucose level is dependent on blood glucose, the CSF glucose level must be evaluated together with the simultaneous blood glucose level (Tülek and Tanyel, 2008).

Bacteriological Investigation

The gold standard diagnostic method for tuberculous meningitis is the culture of the causative agent. CSF should be cultured in at least two different cultures for suspected TBM. Löwenstein-Jensen medium is frequently used for CSF. Today, there are automated systems based on the rapid production of tubercle bacilli, especially MGIT (Mycobacteria Growth Indicator Tube). Even though the time to produce the bacilli in these systems has been reduced to approximately two weeks, this is actually a long time considering the mortal course of the disease. The same automated systems also provide antibiogram susceptibility results within 10 days after the agent is produced.

Molecular Diagnosis

Molecular diagnostic methods in CSF examination are also intensively preferred because traditional methods are difficult and delay in diagnosis. In regions where the disease is endemic, the polymerase chain reaction (PCR) method, which is fast, inexpensive, and has high sensitivity and specificity, is used for early diagnosis (Tunkel et al., 2004).

DNA finger printing, RFLP, MTD ("Amplified M. tuberculosis Direct Test"), and TMA ("Transcription Mediated Amplification") can be used in detailed etiological-diagnostic studies of tuberculous meningitis cases. A number of new molecular methods or combinations of them have been introduced to understand which mycobacterium species develops mycobacterial infections (Jagielski et al., 2014). In the diagnosis of tuberculous meningitis, the demonstration of elevated ADA activity in the CSF is one of the tests that is increasingly used today (Li et al., 2009). In addition, methods such as the detection of tuberculostearic acid, a structural component of mycobacterium, by gas-liquid chromatography, the detection of antibodies against M. tuberculosis antigen-5 by ELISA and the measurement of some neurochemical markers (nitrite, vitamin B12, homocysteine, GABA, tryptophan, taurine, phenylalanine, etc.) are also being developed (Janvier et al., 2010). In order to develop a bacterium-specific antigen and a specific antibody that develops against this antigen, many methods such as hemagglutination (HA), immunofluorescence assay (IFA), radioimmunoassay (RIA) and immunoblot assay have been investigated, but they have not yet entered routine use because their sensitivity and specificity are not yet at the desired level (Turkish Thoracic Society Tuberculosis Study Group, 2019).

Radiological Diagnosis

Computed tomography (CT) and magnetic resonance imaging (MRI) are very useful modalities for visualizing the pathologic changes in the brain due to tuberculous meningitis. In particular, findings such as enlargement of the ventricles, tuberculoma development, abscess formation, infarcts and hydrocephalus development, involvement of the basal regions, and thickening of the meninges can be easily demonstrated. These methods are not pathognomonic in diagnosis. Infarcts can often be seen in the thalamus, basal ganglia, and internal capsule regions. The presence of vasculitis and thrombosis can be detected by radiological methods and may be observed as hypodensity secondary to ischemia on CT. Repeated CT and MRI examinations in the follow-up of patients with tuberculous meningitis make an important contribution both in the diagnosis and in the management of complications. CT is especially useful in the detection of hydrocephalus. MRI is more sensitive in showing meningeal involvement (Kilani et al., 2003).

Treatment

Tuberculous meningitis should be treated with antituberculosis drugs that can pass into the CSF. Initial treatment with at least 3 drugs and maintenance treatment with at least 2 drugs should be combined. Isoniazid, rifampicin, and pyrazinamide should be included in the treatment because they are bactericidal and pass into the CSF. If the incidence of resistance to antituberculosis drugs is above 4%, streptomycin, which has a higher rate of passage into the CSF, should be preferred as the fourth drug. As in pulmonary tuberculosis, the treatment of tuberculous meningitis is recommended as in pulmonary tuberculosis, with 4 drugs for two months in initial treatment and two drugs for 9-12 months in maintenance treatment (Marx and Chan, 2011).

In HIV-positive patients, it is usually sufficient to start treatment with isoniazid, rifampicin, pyrazinamide, and streptomycin for 24 months and then continue with rifampicin and isoniazid for a total of 9-12 months. Ethambutol can be given instead of streptomycin. Unlike other patients, isoniazid is recommended for life after completion of treatment in these patients (Berenguer et al., 1992; McArthur et al., 2005).

Steroid treatment in patients with tuberculous meningitis is still controversial. Studies have shown that steroid treatment improves patients' consciousness, decreases headaches, and improves CSF findings.

In cases of 300 mm/water and above, focal neurologic impairment, altered consciousness, and spinal block, steroid administration is recommended. At the same time, steroid treatment should be given to patients with stage 3, and in stages 1 and 2, steroid treatment should be decided according to the patient's condition. In the initial period, the recommended steroid dose for adult patients is prednisolone 60 mg/day, and in the following period, depending on the clinical status of the patient.

Although it is decided in parallel, it is recommended to be decreased after 1-2 weeks and terminated within 4-6 weeks in total (Haas and Des Perez, 1994).

In the presence of hydrocephalus in patients with tuberculous meningitis, surgical treatment is a treatment option that can sometimes be lifesaving. Ventriculo-peritoneal or ventriculo-atrial shunt operations can be performed. External ventricular drainage can also be performed as a short-term intervention if the patient's condition is appropriate (Molavi and LeFrock, 1985).

Conclusion

Tuberculous meningitis remains a problem with a high mortality rate. Since the diagnosis of the disease is still problematic, the clinical findings of the patients and the tests planned for the diagnosis should be interpreted very carefully. Although the gold standard diagnostic method is bacilli isolation, imaging methods should be utilized in the diagnostic phase.

References

Berenguer, J., Moreno, S., Laguna, F., Vicente, T., Adrados, M., Ortega, A., & Bouza, E. (1992). Tuberculous meningitis in patients infected with the human immunodeficiency virus. *New England Journal of Medicine,* 326(10), 668-672. https://doi.org/10.1056/NEJM199203053261004.

Bonsu, B. K., & Harper, M. B. (2005). Accuracy and test characteristics of ancillary tests of cerebrospinal fluid for predicting acute bacterial meningitis in children with low white blood cell count in cerebrospinal fluid. *Academic emergency medicine,* 12(4), 303-309. https://doi.org/10.1197/j.aem.2004.11.022.

Chan, K. H., Cheung, R. T. F., Lee, R., Mak, W., & Ho, S. L. (2005). Cerebral infarcts complicating tuberculous meningitis. *Cerebrovascular Diseases*, 19(6), 391-395. https://doi.org/10.1159/000085568.

Cotton, M. F., Donald, P. R., Schoeman, J. F., Aalbers, C., Van Zyl, L. E., & Lombard, C. (1991). Plasma arginine vasopressin and the syndrome of inappropriate antidiuretic hormone secretion in tuberculous meningitis. *The Pediatric infectious disease journal*, 10(11), 837-842. https://doi.org/10.1097/00006454-199111000-00009.

Dastur, D. K., Manghani, D. K., & Udani, P. M. (1995). Pathology and pathogenetic mechanisms in neurotuberculosis. *Radiologic Clinics of North America*, 33(4), 733-752. https://doi.org/10.1016/S0033-8389(22)00616-9.

Donald, P. R., Schaaf, H. S., & Schoeman, J. F. (2005). Tuberculous meningitis and miliary tuberculosis: the Rich focus revisited. *Journal of Infection*, 50(3), 193-195. https://doi.org/10.1016/j.jinf.2004.02.010.

Ellard, G. A., Humphries, M. J., Gabriel, M., & Teoh, R. (1987). Penetration of pyrazinamide into the cerebrospinal fluid in tuberculous meningitis. *British medical journal (Clinical research ed.)*, 294(6567), 284. https://doi.org/10.1136/bmj.294.6567.284.

Gray, L. D., & Fedorko, D. P. (1992). Laboratory diagnosis of bacterial meningitis. *Clinical microbiology reviews,* 5(2), 130-145. https://doi.org/10.1128/cmr.5.2.130.

Gupta, R. K., & Kumar, S. (2011). Central nervous system tuberculosis. *Neuroimaging Clinics*, 21(4), 795-814. https://doi.org/10.1016/j.nic.2011.07.004.

Haas, D. W., & Des Prez, R. M. (1994). Tuberculosis and acquired immunodeficiency syndrome: a historical perspective on recent developments. *The American journal of medicine*, 96(5), 439-450. https://doi.org/10.1016/0002-9343(94)90171-6.

Jagielski, T., Van Ingen, J., Rastogi, N., Dziadek, J., Mazur, P. K., & Bielecki, J. (2014). Current methods in the molecular typing of Mycobacterium tuberculosis and other mycobacteria. *BioMed research international,* 2014. https://doi.org/10.1155/2014/645802.

Janvier, F., Servonnet, A., Delacour, H., Fontan, E., Ceppa, E., & Burnat, P. (2010). Interêt du dosage de l'adénosine désaminase dans les infections tuberculeuses neuroméningées [Interest of adenosine deaminase assay in neuromeningeal tuberculosis infections.]. *Med Trop*, 70, 88-93.

Joint Tuberculosis Committee of the British Thoracic Society. (1998). Chemotherapy and management of tuberculosis in the United Kingdom: recommendations 1998. *Thorax*, 53(7), 536-548. http://dx.doi.org/10.1136/thx.53.7.536.

Kanra, G. (1993). Bacterial Meningitis. In: Kanra, G., Akalın, H. E. (Editors). *Infectious Diseases Approach to Acute Bacterial Infections* (44-65). Ankara: Güneş Publishing House.

Kasik, J. E. (1994). Central nervous system tuberculosis. In *Tuberculosis* (pp. 129-142). New York, NY: Springer New York. https://doi.org/10.1007/978-1-4613-8321-5_12.

Katti, M. K. (2004). Pathogenesis, diagnosis, treatment, and outcome aspects of cerebral tuberculosis. *Medical science monitor: international medical journal of experimental and clinical research*, 10(9), RA215-29. PMID: 15328498.

Kent, S. J., Crowe, S. M., Yung, A., Lucas, C. R., & Mijch, A. M. (1993). Tuberculous meningitis: a 30-year review. *Clinical infectious diseases*, 17(6), 987-994. https://doi.org/10.1093/clinids/17.6.987.

Kilani, B., Ammari, L., Tiouiri, H., Goubontini, A., Kanoun, F., Zouiten, F., & Chaabène, T. B. (2003). Manifestations neuroradiologiques initiales de la tuberculose du système nerveux central de l'adulte [Neuroradiologic manifestations of central nervous system tuberculosis in 122 adults]. À propos de 122 cas. *La Revue de médecine interne,* 24(2), 86-96. https://doi.org/10.1016/S0248-8663(02)00716-6.

Leonard, J. M. (2017). Central nervous system tuberculosis. *Tuberculosis and nontuberculous mycobacterial infections,* 331-341. https://doi.org/10.1128/9781555819866.ch20.

Lewinsohn, D. M., Leonard, M. K., LoBue, P. A., Cohn, D. L., Daley, C. L., Desmond, E., Keane, J., Lewinsohn, D. A., Loeffler, A. M., Mazurek, G. H., O'Brien, R. J., Pai, M., Richeldi, L., Salfinger, M., Shinnick, T. M., Sterling, T. R., Warshauer, D. M., & Woods, G. L. (2017). Official American Thoracic Society/Infectious Diseases Society of America/Centers for Disease Control and Prevention clinical practice guidelines: diagnosis of tuberculosis in adults and children. *Clinical Infectious Diseases,* 64(2), e1-e33. https://doi.org/10.1093/cid/ciw694.

Li, H., Turhan, V., Chokhani, L., Stratton, C. W., Dunbar, S. A., & Tang, Y. W. (2009). Identification and differentiation of clinically relevant mycobacterium species directly from acid-fast bacillus-positive culture broth. *Journal of clinical microbiology*, 47(12), 3814-3820. https://doi.org/10.1128/jcm.01534-09.

Marx, G. E., & Chan, E. D. (2011). Tuberculous meningitis: diagnosis and treatment overview. *Tuberculosis research and treatment,* 2011, 1-9. https://doi.org/10.1155/2011/798764.

McArthur, J. C., Brew, B. J., & Nath, A. (2005). Neurological complications of HIV infection. *The Lancet Neurology,* 4(9), 543-555. https://doi.org/10.1016/S1474-4422(05)70165-4.

Mezochow, A., Thakur, K., & Vinnard, C. (2017). Tuberculous meningitis in children and adults: new insights for an ancient foe. *Current neurology and neuroscience reports,* 17, 1-12. https://doi.org/10.1007/s11910-017-0796-0.

Molavi, A., & LeFrock, J. L. (1985). Tuberculous meningitis. *The Medical clinics of North America,* 69(2), 315-331. https://doi.org/10.1016/s0025-7125(16)31045-8.

Roca, B. (2005). Intradural extramedullary tuberculoma of the spinal cord: a review of reported cases. *Journal of Infection*, 50(5), 425-431. https://doi.org/10.1016/j.jinf.2004.07.012.

Sheller, J. R., & Prez, R. M. D. (1986). CNS tuberculosis. *Neurologic clinics*, 4(1), 143-158. https://doi.org/10.1016/S0733-8619(18)30992-7.

Thwaites, G. E., & Hien, T. T. (2005). Tuberculous meningitis: many questions, too few answers. *The Lancet Neurology*, 4(3), 160-170. https://doi.org/10.1016/S1474-4422(05)01013-6.

Tülek, N. & Tanyel, E. (2008). Overview of Central Nervous System Infections. In: Topçu, W. A., Söyletir, G., Doğanay, M. (Editors). *Infectious Diseases and Microbiology* (pp. 1375-1390). Istanbul: Nobel Medicine Publisher.

Tülek, N., & Fışkın, N. T. (2008) Acute Bacterial Meningitis. In: Topçu, A. W., Söyletir, G., Doğanay, M. (Editors). *Infectious Diseases and Microbiology* (1390-1422). Istanbul: Nobel Medicine Publisher.

Tunkel, A. R., Hartman, B. J., Kaplan, S. L., Kaufman, B. A., Roos, K. L., Scheld, W. M., & Whitley, R. J. (2004). Practice guidelines for the management of bacterial meningitis. *Clinical infectious diseases,* 39(9), 1267-1284. https://doi.org/10.1086/425368.

Turkish Thoracic Society Tuberculosis Study Group (2019). *Tuberculosis* (3-13). Ankara, Turkish Thoracic Society Educational Books Series. [Internet]. [cite 25 July 2023]. https://toraks.org.tr/site/sf/documents/pre_migration/573e1a496aeb0e3828490055e403108860b2949dd6691fa67a6198b03d930bc2.pdf.

van den Bos, F., Terken, M., Ypma. L., Kimpen, J. L., Nel, E. D., Schaaf, H. S., Schoeman, J. F., Donald, P. R. (2004). Tuberculous meningitis and miliary tuberculosis in young children. *Trop Med Int Health,* 9(2):309-313. https://doi.org/10.1046/j.1365-3156.2003.01185.x.

WHO (2019). *Global Tuberculosis Report.* Geneva: World Health Organization; 2019.

Chapter 7

Encephalomyelitis and Neuritis

Bahadır O. Özbay*, MD
Department of Infectious Diseases and Clinical Microbiology, Tokat State Hospital, Tokat, Turkiye

Abstract

Encephalomyelitis is a rare syndrome that is often overlooked at diagnosis. Acute disseminated encephalomyelitis (ADEM) is an autoimmune demyelinating central nervous system disease that typically follows an infection. The typical presentation is with an acute onset of multifocal neurological symptoms and rapid worsening, often leading to hospitalization. In patients, the results of cerebrospinal fluid analysis are variable. Lymphocytic pleocytosis and a mild increase in protein can be seen as findings in cerebrospinal fluid analysis. Magnetic resonance imaging is the main imaging modality in patients with suspected ADEM. Multiple sclerosis is at the first place in the differential diagnosis of ADEM. The main treatment for ADEM is immunosuppressive therapy. Tumors are detected in some of the patients diagnosed with encephalomyelitis (paraneoplastic encephalomyelitis). The most common accompanying tumor of paraneoplastic encephalomyelitis is small cell lung cancer. The clinical manifestations of encephalomyelitis depend on the CNS regions involved. Tumor resection and chemotherapy can be started, as well as steroids, intravenous immunoglobulins, or plasmapheresis treatment. Optic neuritis is an inflammation of the optic nerve that often causes temporary loss of vision. The most common cause of optic neuritis is multiple sclerosis. Other optic neuropathies may be associated with various infectious diseases.

---

* Corresponding Author's Email: orkun-ozbay@hotmail.com.

In: Central Nervous System Infections
Editor: Mustafa Usanmaz
ISBN: 979-8-89113-660-1

Keywords: encephalomyelitis, encephalitis, neuritis, acute disseminated encephalomyelitis, optic neuritis

Introduction

Encephalomyelitis is inflammation of the brain parenchyma and spinal cord caused by autoimmune or viral infections. Acute disseminated encephalomyelitis (ADEM) is an inflammatory demyelinating disease of the central nervous system that affects the brain and spinal cord. Tumors are detected in some patients with autoimmune encephalomyelitis (paraneoplastic encephalomyelitis). The clinical findings of encephalomyelitis may differ according to the region involved in the central nervous system. Encephalomyelitis is a rare syndrome that is often overlooked at diagnosis. Optic neuritis is the neuritis best described in relation to infectious agents. It has also been described in the post-vaccination period.

Encephalomyelitis

Acute Disseminated encephalomyelitis (ADEM)

Acute disseminated encephalomyelitis (ADEM) is an inflammatory demyelinating disease of the central nervous system (CNS) that affects the brain and spinal cord. ADEM is an autoimmune demyelinating central nervous system disease that typically follows an infection. ADEM is also known as post-infectious encephalomyelitis. Its pathogenesis is not fully understood, but it is thought to be an autoimmune disease that occurs after an environmental trigger, such as viral infections. In pathogenesis, it is thought that an autoimmune reaction develops because myelin auto antigens contain a common antigenic determinant with the infecting pathogen (Garg, 2003). The most important histopathological finding is perivenous demyelination and lymphocyte and macrophage infiltration.

ADEM is generally considered a post- or parainfectious disease. In the adult patient group, the rate of previous infection was 50-75% in patients with ADEM (Ketelslegers et al., 2011; Koelman et al., 2016). We can list the infectious pathogens associated with ADEM as follows: measles, rubella, mumps, varicella, influenza, cytomegalovirus, Epstein-Barr virus, herpes simplex virus, human herpes virus-6, HIV, mycoplasma pneumonia, group a streptococcus, borrelia burgdorferi, and leptospira (Dale et al., 2001; Denes et al., 2004; Hart & Earle, 1975; Kaji et al., 1996; Silver et al., 1997; Tsiodras et al., 2006). There have also been a few reported cases of ADEM after severe acute respiratory syndrome coronavirus 2 (SARS-CoV-2) infection (Parsons et al., 2020). Post-vaccine encephalomyelitis accounts for a small portion of ADEM cases.

ADEM is more common in childhood than in the adult age group. The incidence decreased after vaccination became widespread, but it still occurs. The median age in studies reported in adults is between 33 and 37 years (Koelman et al., 2016). In adult patients, no significant differences were found between genders.

Acute disseminated encephalomyelitis is usually a monophasic disease. The typical presentation is with an acute onset of multifocal neurological symptoms (accompanied by encephalopathy) and rapid worsening, often leading to hospitalization. In some cases, systemic symptoms such as fever, malaise, myalgia, and headache can be seen in the initial period. Change of consciousness, pyramidal tract findings, ataxia, cranial nerve involvement, and optic neuritis are frequently observed. A wide range of symptoms present within the neurological spectrum, consciousness is normal or may be in the range leading to coma. In addition, multifocal neurological disorders such as aphasia, motor and sensory deficits, movement disorders and meningism, and symptoms of acute meningoencephalopathy, seizures, and psychosis may be seen. The presence of encephalopathy in adults is important in the differential diagnosis to distinguish it from other diseases (e.g., multiple sclerosis). Acute hemorrhagicencephalomyelitis (AHEM), which is considered a rare variant of ADEM, is a hyperacute variant with hemorrhages that can progress rapidly (Hart & Earle, 1975). Neuroimaging usually shows hemorrhagic lesions in the white matter.

CSF analysis should be performed by lumbar puncture in patients with suspected ADEM. In patients, CSF analysis results are variable. The CSF findings may be normal in some patients. Abnormal CSF results can be detected in 50-80% of patients (Höllinger et al., 2002; Schwarz et al., 2001). Lymphocytic pleocytosis and a mild increase in protein can be seen as findings in the CSF analysis. Although not as common as in MS, oligoclonal bands can also be detected in ADEM. In addition, in patients with suspected ADEM, anti-myelin oligodendrocyteglycoprotein (MOG)-IgG and anti-aquaporin-4-IgG autoantibodies with serological tests may be helpful in diagnosis (López-Chiriboga et al., 2018).

Computed tomography (CT) of the brain is usually normal or non-diagnostic, especially in the early stages of ADEM. Magnetic resonance imaging (MRI) is the main imaging modality in patients with suspected ADEM. In patients with suspected ADEM, in addition to brain MRI, cervical and thoracic spine MRI should also be performed if there are signs and symptoms of myelopathy. MRI images may be normal during the patient's admission to the hospital. Cases of MRI abnormalities have been reported 5-14 days after the onset of symptoms. Therefore, in the clinical picture of the patient ADEM suspected, but pathological finding on MRI is not detected, this should be taken into account. The acute MRI features of the disseminated encephalomyelitis could be defined in more detail. Lesions are usually large, asymmetrical, often multiple, and are always bilateral. The distributed locations of the lesions are quite different. Lesions are slightly hypointense with large ones on T1-weighted sequences and hyperintense on T2-weighted and fluid-attenuated inversion-healing (FLAIR) sequences (Singh et al., 1999). In addition, the enhancement of gadolinium in lesions is generally variable (Schwarz et al., 2001). The electroencephalogram (EEG) in ADEM has been studied, but the findings are often non-specific. It usually does not contribute to the diagnosis. There is no consensus on diagnostic criteria for ADEM in adults.

Multiple sclerosis (MS) is at the forefront of the differential diagnosis of ADEM. It is difficult to distinguish between MS and ADEM in adults. There is usually a history of viral infection before ADEM, but not in MS. ADEM usually produces a more diffuse central nervous system disorder, whereas MS is typically monosymptomatic. ADEM has more bilateral, asymmetric, white matter abnormalities compared to early MS. Infectious meningoencephalitis, neurosarcoidosis, vasculitis, progressive multifocal leukoencephalopathy, and Behçet's syndrome are other diseases in the differential diagnosis.

The main treatment for ADEM is immunosuppressive therapy. First-line treatment for patients diagnosed with ADEM, a high dose (1000 mg daily) intravenous methylprednisolone is started for 3-5 days (Schwarz et al., 2001). Afterwards, maintenance dose therapy with steroid is continued. In case of insufficient response to treatment plasmapheresis or intravenous immunoglobulins (IVIG) can be considered as an option (Marchioni et al., 2002).

Most patients with mild symptoms improve with treatment or spontaneously (Marchioni et al., 2002). Mortality rates have been reported to be more than 20% in historical studies (Gibbons et al., 1956), but mortality rates have been reported at a lower rate (4-12%) in more recent studies (Ketelslegers et al., 2011; Schwarz et al., 2001).

Paraneoplastic Encephalomyelitis

Encephalomyelitis is mostly viral or autoimmune, occurring due to causes. Tumors are detected in some patients diagnosed with encephalomyelitis. Tumors can cause encephalomyelitis by autoimmune mechanisms. The most common accompanying tumor of paraneoplastic encephalomyelitis is small cell lung cancer. Encephalomyelitis other types of cancer reported in cases of lymphoma, esophagus, breast, ovary, pancreas, liver, and kidney cancers and germ cell tumors (Galli & Greenlee, 2020). Effective early recognition of the clinical syndrome for treatment by demonstrating the underlying tumor and accompanying antibodies. It is important to quickly elucidate the paraneoplastic ethology. In most cases of paraneoplastic encephalomyelitis, neurological findings go beyond the diagnosis of cancer. Cancer manifestations are often 4-12 months after the onset of neurological signs emerges in. The clinical manifestations of encephalomyelitis depend on the CNS regions involved (Dalmau et al., 1992). However, in most cases of encephalomyelitis, epileptic seizures, altered consciousness, behavior change, short-term memory loss, extrapyramidal and autonomic findings are detected. Tumor resection and chemotherapy can be started, as well as steroids, IVIG or plasmapheresis treatment. Immunosuppressive agents from one to the other there is no scientific evidence to show that it is superior.

Neuritis

Optic Neuritis

Optic neuritis is an inflammation of the optic nerve that often causes temporary loss of vision. The underlying pathogenic factor often triggers demyelinating processes. Typically, it occurs acutely and shows unilateral involvement. The most common cause of optic neuritis is multiple sclerosis. Atypical optic neuritis may be characterized by bilateral involvement and may also have systemic symptoms. Atypical optic neurpathies may be associated with various infectious diseases (Table 1) (Kahloun et al., 2015). There are different opinions about the pathogenesis of infectious optic neuropathies. There may be direct involvement of the optic nerve by a pathogen. There may have been indirect optic nerve involvement by inflammatory, degenerative, or vascular mechanisms. Infectious agents can cause optic neuritis, as well as ethambutol, isoniazid, chloramphenicol, and sulfonamides can cause optic neuritis as a side effect. Optic nerve involvement has also been described in association with vaccination. Post-vaccination optic neuritis can occur hours to weeks later. It is thought to be an immune-mediated mechanism in its pathogenesis. Optic neuropathy has been reported after Bacillus Calmette-Guérin vaccine, influenza virus, hepatitis B virus, hepatitis A virus, yellow fever, measles/rubella vaccines, mumps, diphtheria toxoid, tetanus toxoid, rabies virus, and variola virus vaccination (Kahloun et al., 2015).

Table 1. Infectious agents causing optic neuropathies

Bacterial
Borrelia burgdorferi (Lyme disease)
Bartonella henselae (Cat-scratch disease)
Treponema pallidum (Syphilis)
Mycobacterium tuberculosis (Tuberculosis)
Coxiella burnetii (Q fever)
Tropheryma whippleii (Whipple disease)
Brucellosis
Rickettsioses
Viral
West Nile
Dengue fever
Chikungunya
Herpes simplex 1 and 2
Varicella-Zoster
Cytomegalovirus
Epstein-Barr
Measles
Mumps
Rubella
Influenza
Parasitic
Toxoplasma gondii (Toxoplasmosis)
Toxocara canis (Toxocariasis)
Fungal
Cryptococcus neoformans (Cryptococcus)
Aspergillus fumigatus (Aspergillus)

Conclusion

Encephalomyelitis and neuritis can be seen due to infectious causes. It can also be seen due to vaccinations. Immune mechanisms play a role in the pathogenesis of encephalomyelitis and neuritis. Accurate and rapid diagnosis and early treatment lead to better outcomes. An important part of treatment is immunosuppressive therapy.

References

Dale, R. C., Church, A. J., Cardoso, F., Goddard, E., Cox, T. C., Chong, W. K., Williams, A., Klein, N. J., Neville, B. G., Thompson, E. J., & Giovannoni, G. (2001). Poststreptococcal acute disseminated encephalomyelitis with basal ganglia involvement and auto-reactive antibasal ganglia antibodies. *Ann Neurol*, *50*(5), 588-595. https://doi.org/10.1002/ana.1250.

Dalmau, J., Graus, F., Rosenblum, M. K., & Posner, J. B. (1992). Anti-Hu--associated paraneoplastic encephalomyelitis/sensory neuronopathy. A clinical study of 71 patients. *Medicine (Baltimore)*, *71*(2), 59-72. https://doi.org/10.1097/00005792-199203000-00001.

Denes, E., Magy, L., Pradeau, K., Alain, S., Weinbreck, P., & Ranger-Rogez, S. (2004). Successful treatment of human herpesvirus 6 encephalomyelitis in immunocompetent patient. *Emerg Infect Dis*, *10*(4), 729-731. https://doi.org/10.3201/eid1004.030587.

Galli, J., & Greenlee, J. (2020). Paraneoplastic Diseases of the Central Nervous System. *F1000Res*, *9*. https://doi.org/10.12688/f1000research.21309.1.

Garg, R. K. (2003). Acute disseminated encephalomyelitis. *Postgrad Med J*, *79*(927), 11-17. https://doi.org/10.1136/pmj.79.927.11.

Gibbons, J. L., Miller, H. G., & Stanton, J. B. (1956). Para-infectious encephalomyelitis and related syndromes; a critical review of the neurological complications of certain specific fevers. *Q J Med,* 25(100), 427-505.

Hart, M. N., & Earle, K. M. (1975). Haemorrhagic and perivenous encephalitis: a clinical-pathological review of 38 cases. *J Neurol Neurosurg Psychiatry*, *38*(6), 585-591. https://doi.org/10.1136/jnnp.38.6.585.

Höllinger, P., Sturzenegger, M., Mathis, J., Schroth, G., & Hess, C. W. (2002). Acute disseminated encephalomyelitis in adults: a reappraisal of clinical, CSF, EEG, and MRI findings. *J Neurol*, *249*(3), 320-329. https://doi.org/10.1007/s004150200012.

Kahloun, R., Abroug, N., Ksiaa, I., Mahmoud, A., Zeghidi, H., Zaouali, S., & Khairallah, M. (2015). Infectious optic neuropathies: a clinical update. *Eye Brain*, *7*, 59-81. https://doi.org/10.2147/eb.s69173.

Kaji, M., Kusuhara, T., Ayabe, M., Hino, H., Shoji, H., & Nagao, T. (1996). Survey of herpes simplex virus infections of the central nervous system, including acute disseminated encephalomyelitis, in the Kyushu and Okinawa regions of Japan. *Mult Scler*, *2*(2), 83-87. https://doi.org/10.1177/135245859600200204.

Ketelslegers, I. A., Visser, I. E., Neuteboom, R. F., Boon, M., Catsman-Berrevoets, C. E., & Hintzen, R. Q. (2011). Disease course and outcome of acute disseminated encephalomyelitis is more severe in adults than in children. *Mult Scler*, *17*(4), 441-448. https://doi.org/10.1177/1352458510390068.

Koelman, D. L., Chahin, S., Mar, S. S., Venkatesan, A., Hoganson, G. M., Yeshokumar, A. K., Barreras, P., Majmudar, B., Klein, J. P., Chitnis, T., Benkeser, D. C., Carone, M., & Mateen, F. J. (2016). Acute disseminated encephalomyelitis in 228 patients: A retrospective, multicenter US study. *Neurology*, 86(22), 2085-2093. https://doi.org/10.1212/wnl.0000000000002723.

López-Chiriboga, A. S., Majed, M., Fryer, J., Dubey, D., McKeon, A., Flanagan, E. P., Jitprapaikulsan, J., Kothapalli, N., Tillema, J. M., Chen, J., Weinshenker, B., Wingerchuk, D., Sagen, J., Gadoth, A., Lennon, V. A., Keegan, B. M., Lucchinetti, C., & Pittock, S. J. (2018). Association of MOG-IgG Serostatus With Relapse After Acute Disseminated Encephalomyelitis and Proposed Diagnostic Criteria for MOG-IgG-Associated Disorders. *JAMA Neurol*, *75*(11), 1355-1363. https://doi.org/10.1001/jamaneurol.2018.1814.

Marchioni, E., Marinou-Aktipi, K., Uggetti, C., Bottanelli, M., Pichiecchio, A., Soragna, D., PiccoloG, Imbesi, F., Romani, A., & Ceroni, M. (2002). Effectiveness of intravenous immunoglobulin treatment in adult patients with steroid-resistant monophasic or recurrent acute disseminated encephalomyelitis. *J Neurol*, *249*(1), 100-104. https://doi.org/10.1007/pl00007836.

Parsons, T., Banks, S., Bae, C., Gelber, J., Alahmadi, H., & Tichauer, M. (2020). COVID-19-associated acute disseminated encephalomyelitis (ADEM). *J Neurol*, *267*(10), 2799-2802. https://doi.org/10.1007/s00415-020-09951-9.

Schwarz, S., Mohr, A., Knauth, M., Wildemann, B., & Storch-Hagenlocher, B. (2001). Acute disseminated encephalomyelitis: a follow-up study of 40 adult patients. *Neurology*, *56*(10), 1313-1318. https://doi.org/10.1212/wnl.56.10.1313.

Silver, B., McAvoy, K., Mikesell, S., & Smith, T. W. (1997). Fulminating encephalopathy with perivenular demyelination and vacuolar myelopathy as the initial presentation of human immunodeficiency virus infection. *Arch Neurol*, *54*(5), 647-650. https://doi.org/10.1001/archneur.1997.00550170115023.

Singh, S., Alexander, M., & Korah, I. P. (1999). Acute disseminated encephalomyelitis: MR imaging features. *AJR Am J Roentgenol*, *173*(4), 1101-1107. https://doi.org/10.2214/ajr.173.4.10511187.

Tsiodras, S., Kelesidis, T., Kelesidis, I., Voumbourakis, K., & Giamarellou, H. (2006). Mycoplasma pneumoniae-associated myelitis: a comprehensive review. *Eur J Neurol*, *13*(2), 112-124. https://doi.org/10.1111/j.1468-1331.2006.01174.x.

Chapter 8

Epidural Abscess, Subdural Empyema, and Brain Abscess

Arzu Altuncekic Yildirim*, MD
Department of Infectious Diseases and Clinical Microbiology, Ordu University, Ordu, Turkiye

Abstract

Central nervous system (CNS) infections are infections that progress rapidly and have high morbidity and mortality. Various causative agents, including viruses, bacteria, fungi, protozoa, and helminths, can infect the CNS. Infection can develop in the cranial area or spinal column. The presence of various factors, such as different clinical presentations, the virulence of the causative agent, and the affected area, makes the diagnosis challenging. Hence, providing rapid treatment approaches in clinically suspicious patients is important for their chance of survival. Epidural abscess, subdural empyema, and brain abscess will be discussed among CNS infections in this chapter.

Keywords: epidural abscess, subdural empyema, brain abscess

Introduction

Epidural abscess, subdural empyema, and brain abscess are severe and potentially life-threatening infections of the central nervous system. Although its overall incidence decreases, there are high-risk patient populations with

* Corresponding Author's Email: arzaltu@gmail.com.

In: Central Nervous System Infections
Editor: Mustafa Usanmaz
ISBN: 979-8-89113-660-1

penetrating head trauma, neurosurgery, or a history of immunodeficiency. They require a multidisciplinary approach. Quick diagnosis and treatment are essential due to the high risk of morbidity and mortality associated with possible complications.

Epidural Abscess

Epidural abscess represents a localized collection of pus between the dura mater and the overlying skull or vertebral column. It can occur intracranially (intracranial epidural abscess), but more often in the space between the bones of the spine and the spinal cord (spinal epidural abscess) (Akhondi and Baker, 2022). The dura mater forms the inner lining of the skull, and there is usually no space between the skull and the dura. Increased intracranial pressure due to infections, inflammation, or tumors opens the epidural space and separates bone from tissue. Epidural abscesses occur as a result of infections that affect the *spinal or cranial* epidural space. Intracranial epidural abscesses (IEA) may develop as a complication of sinusitis and otitis. Nowadays, the frequency of these infections has decreased with more effective treatment. However, they may develop secondary to cranial surgery or trauma.

Spinal epidural abscess (SEA) is observed more frequently than IEA (Reihsaus et al., 2000). It may be acute or chronic. Whereas the incidence of SEA has been reported as 2 cases per 10,000 hospitalizations, there have been centers reporting this rate as 10/10000 in recent years (Artenstein et al., 2016). The elderly population with comorbidities, the increase in intravenous (iv) drug use and surgical procedures, and the more widespread use of diagnostic imaging methods are thought to be effective in this increase in rate. Diabetes, iv drug use, chronic kidney failure, alcoholism, or immunosuppression are among the risk factors.

Pathophysiologically, it can occur as contiguous or hematogenous. The spread of infections such as vertebral osteomyelitis and discitis, penetrating injuries, surgical or spinal interventions, and procedures such as a lumbar puncture or paravertebral injection may be the source of it. The presence of an intravenous catheter, the use of drugs by injection, or the presence of endocarditis are important risk factors in cases of SEA developing hematogenously. In 25-50% of patients, it develops secondary to infections such as skin soft tissue infections, urinary infections, periodontal abscesses, pneumonia, and mastoiditis.

Most epidural abscesses are polymicrobial. They include anaerobic gram-positive cocci, staphylococci, streptococci, and anaerobic gram-negative bacilli. Anaerobic organisms are especially important in sinusitis-related epidural abscesses.

S. *aureus* is the responsible microorganism in SEA at a rate of 50-90%. Aerobic and anaerobic *streptococci* and gram-negative bacilli, particularly *E. coli* and *Pseudomonas*, are other possible agents. Intravenous drug use is a significant risk for *Pseudomonas*. *Nocardia* and *Actinomyces* have been reported as causative agents in case reports (Martínez de Pinillos Sánchez et al., 2022; Kapmaz et al., 2014). In countries where tuberculosis and brucellosis constitute a problem, they should be considered causative agents.

Clinically, the findings in IEA are usually insidious because the abscess progresses slowly. In the case of co-existence, it can be evaluated as a complaint of otitis or sinusitis. Acute neurological deficits can manifest themselves with focal or generalized seizures. About 45% of patients also have periorbital cellulitis or frontal edema. Papilledema and other signs of increased intracranial pressure develop in untreated patients as the abscess enlarges. Cranial nerve involvement and focal neurological deficits may also develop.

The presentation of SEA progresses in four clinical stages in most patients. First, back pain and focal vertebral pain with tenderness, nerve root pain manifested by radiculopathy or paresthesia or both, spinal cord dysfunction characterized by defects in motor, sensory, or sphincter functions, and paraplegia are observed on examination. Neurological symptoms depend on the level of spinal cord involvement. Local tenderness at the affected level usually accompany them. Pain becomes severe as the infection progresses. It is very important to suspect SEA before the onset of neurological deficits in patients with back pain. Although there are series reporting fever at 60-70%, it may not accompany them, especially in chronic processes (Davis et al., 2004).

Laboratory findings are nonspecific in the diagnosis. Especially high levels of CRP in the beginning are important in patients with compatible clinical findings. They will also help evaluate treatment response. A normal white blood cell (WBC) count does not exclude it. Blood cultures must be obtained prior to initiating empirical antibiotic therapy. Positivity reaching 59% is reported in monomicrobial etiology (Sobottke et al.,2010). Gadolinium-enriched magnetic resonance imaging (MRI) is a preferred method in imaging. MRI allows differential diagnosis with other intracranial pathologies. Additionally, it can identify accompanying osteomyelitis, intramedullary spinal cord lesions, and discitis. It is possible to distinguish sterile effusion and hematoma with gadolinium involvement (Ren et al., 2023).

Appropriate antimicrobial therapy should be initiated, and surgical drainage should be provided during treatment. Although conservative approaches, including treatment with antibiotics without surgery, have recently been preferred, a high failure rate has been reported (Shah et al.,2018; Schwab and Shah, 2020). On the other hand, advanced age and comorbid factors in many patients increase the surgical risk. Therefore, there is a need for algorithms that will provide the answer to the question of which patient can be treated with a safe conservative treatment. Hunter et al. reported a failure of 36% with conservative treatment (Hunter et al., 2021). Concerning failure, they indicated that infection with *S. aureus*, multifocal involvement, the presence of leucocytosis in the beginning, and neurological deficit were predictive factors. Empirical treatment must be initiated immediately after blood culture is taken. Empirical antibiotic therapy should be in combination with an effective antistaphylococcal agent and gram-negative aerobic microorganisms, particularly in patients addicted to iv drugs and with a history of surgical intervention. The treatment can be modified according to the growth and sensitivity detected in the samples taken with a surgical or interventional procedure. The treatment duration is usually 4-6 weeks, and this period should be extended to 8 weeks if osteomyelitis is present. The recommended duration is 12 months in cases of spondylitis and epidural abscess due to tuberculosis.

Subdural Empyema

Subdural empyema (SE) represents the accumulation of pus in the space between the dura and the arachnoid membrane. It is reported with a frequency of 15-25% among intracranial infections. The mortality rate, which was almost 100% in the past, has decreased considerably with advances in diagnosis and treatment methods today. Due to the absence of an anatomical barrier, subdural empyema may spread to the convexity of the brain between the cerebral hemispheres and the opposite hemisphere, even the posterior fossa in some cases (Fernández-de Thomas and De Jesus,2022). Previous cranial surgery, cranial traumas involving an open fracture or penetrating injury, infected hematoma or subdural effusion, and improperly treated ear and sinus infections can be listed among predisposing conditions. It is reported that 20-

40% of the cases have upper respiratory tract infections, particularly sinusitis, and approximately 20% have cranial injury or surgery (Silverberg and Di Nubile, 1985; Wu et al., 2008). *Streptococci, Staphylococci, Haemophilus influenzae, Streptococcus pneumoniae,* and other gram-negative bacilli are the most common microorganisms in the etiology. The expected frequency of causative agents varies according to the underlying pathology. In SE developing secondary to paranasal sinusitis, anaerobic and microaerophilic streptococci, *Staphylococcus aureus* in cases secondary to skull trauma or surgical procedures, Coagulase-negative *staphylococci*, anaerobes, and gram-negative organisms after trauma or surgical procedures should be considered primarily. Most cases are polymicrobial. There are also reports of unusual causative agents such as S*almonella* (Lu et al., 2022), P*ropionibacterium* (So et al., 2018), M*ycobacterium tuberculosis* (Abdallah, 2021), and C*andida* (Carter, 2008).

SE usually develops as a result of the spread of a local infection. Mastoid or ear infections can spread easily due to venous vessels without valves in cases of epidural abscess and associated osteomyelitis, or thrombophlebitis-associated infection. It can also develop after surgery with direct contaminations during cranial surgery. In infants, it can develop as a complication of purulent meningitis due to infection of sterile, reactive subdural effusions secondary to meningitis.

The clinical picture of SE includes signs of a combination of increased intracranial pressure, meningeal irritation, and the presence of focal inflammation. It should be considered while diagnosing patients with acute bacterial sinusitis along with severe headache, altered state of consciousness, focal neurological deficit, or meningeal irritation signs. Headaches and mental changes are usually accompanied by a fever of 39 degrees or higher. These three clinical findings are less common in children. Focal neurological symptoms may begin within 24-48 hours in cases in which treatment is not initiated. The most common neurological symptoms include hemiparesis, hemiplegia, cranial nerve involvement, and anisocoria. Focal or generalized seizures may develop.

Lumbar puncture for CSF analysis is contraindicated because of increased intracranial pressure and the risk of cerebral herniation. All patients with suspected subdural empyema must undergo cranial imaging. Contrast-enhanced computed tomography (CT) or MRI are the imaging modalities to be selected. It can be detected in existing pathologies such as sinusitis and otitis. On CT, SE appears as a crescent or elliptical hypodense area on the cerebral hemisphere or along the falx. Small collections and localizations that are difficult to detect with CT can be better identified, particularly with gadolinium MRI. Magnetic resonance imaging is more specific to better define the anatomical location, visualize the posterior fossa, and differentiate empyema effusion. Diffusion-weighted images increase the diagnostic value of MRI and provide the distinction of effusion empyema.

SE is an emergency requiring a combined medical and surgical approach. It is necessary to initiate antimicrobial agents and provide abscess drainage. The surgical approach will ensure sample collection for microbiological diagnostic tests and control the increase in intracranial pressure. Gram staining examination, which can be performed in a short time with the supply of purulent material, is a guide for empirical treatment. A combination of third- or fourth-generation cephalosporin and metronidazole or alternatively meropenem can be started in empirical treatment. When *Staphylococcus aureus* is suspected, vancomycin should be started empirically, and antibiotic therapy should be modified with culture results (Sanford, 2023). Linezolid has been used successfully in isolated subdural empyema cases caused by *streptococci.* It can be considered in patients with subdural empyema caused by gram-positive bacteria, which have failed conventionally (Bennett, 2015). The limits of the treatment period are unclear, and antimicrobial therapy should continue for 3-4 weeks after surgery. The duration of treatment should be extended in the presence of concomitant osteomyelitis. The prognosis is associated with the ability to establish an early diagnosis. The prognosis is better in cases in which the preoperative state of consciousness is not bad, in which rapid interventions are performed, and antibiotic therapy is initiated rapidly. Mortality is high in the group of patients with advanced age, stupor, and coma. Epileptic seizures, cerebritis, cerebral abscess, cerebral edema, cortical venous thrombosis with cerebral venous infarction, cavernous sinus thrombosis, sepsis, hydrocephalus, cranial osteomyelitis of adjacent cranial bones, osteomyelitis of the craniotomy bone flap, and residual neurological deficits can be regarded complications.

Brain Abscess

The brain abscess represents a focal suppurative infection of the brain parenchyma. It begins as a localized area of cerebritis and transforms into a collection of pus surrounded by a well-vascularized capsule. Etiologically, it can develop with the spread of localized infection or through the hematogenous route. Paranasal sinus infections, otitis media, mastoiditis, or dental infections may be the source of the direct local spread. Whereas lower temporal and cerebellar abscesses are usually observed due to otitis and mastoiditis, frontal, ethmoid sinus, and dental infections usually cause abscesses in the frontal lobe. The hematogenous spread usually occurs secondary to lung-related problems such as pulmonary abscesses and empyema in patients with bronchiectasis. Cyanotic congenital heart disease has been found to be associated in most cases. Bacterial endocarditis, skin infections, and pelvic or intra-abdominal infections are also areas that can be a source. Abscesses secondary to bacteremia are generally observed in the area supplied by the middle cerebral artery and as multiple abscess foci. Hence, the focus of infection must be investigated by considering the predisposing factors in multiple brain abscesses, which are thought to be of hematogenous origin. On the other hand, it should be kept in mind that the mentioned pathologies may develop as complications during follow-up.

Before human immunodeficiency virus (HIV) infections, its frequency was estimated at 0.3-1.3/year per 100,000 people. However, the annual number of cases and the diversity of causative agents have increased significantly with HIV. It varies depending on the predisposing condition and is most commonly observed in male patients between the ages of 30-40 among adults. General health services and socioeconomic improvements are thought to reduce its incidence. About 25% of brain abscesses are observed in children. They are common in children with otitis media or cyanotic congenital heart disease, usually between 4 and 7 years of age. While the frequency of autogenic abscesses has decreased over the years, the incidence of posttraumatic and postoperative recurrence has increased. Additionally, the increase in the immunosuppressive patient group is also important in the increased incidence. Overall mortality varies between 8% and 25%, although it has decreased dramatically owing to effective antimicrobial regimens, advances in imaging modalities and surgical techniques. There is a 20-70% incidence of neurological sequelae in surviving patients (Bennett, 2015; Bokhari and Mesfin, 2022). It is important to identify predisposing conditions early in order to reduce mortality and morbidity and predict possible microbiological agents. Some bacteria, fungi, protozoa, or helminths can also be detected among the responsible causative agents, especially in the immunosuppressive group (Table 1).

Table 1. The relationship of predisposant pathology - responsible microorganism (Edited from the reference 21)

Predisposant Pathologies	Frequent Microorganisms
Otitis media or mastoiditis	Streptococci (anaerobic or aerobic), Bacteroides and Prevotella spp., Enterobacteriaceae
Sinusitis (frontoethmoid or sphenoid)	Streptococci, Bacteroides spp., Enterobacteriaceae, Staphylococcus aureus, Haemophilus spp.
Dental infection	Mixed Fusobacterium, Prevotella, Actinomyces, and Bacteroides spp., Streptococci
Penetrating trauma or postneurosurgical	S. aureus, streptococci, Enterobacteriaceae, Clostridium spp
Lung abscess, empyema, bronchiectasis	Fusobacterium, Actinomyces, Bacteroides, and Prevotella spp., Streptococci, Nocardia spp.
Bacterial endocarditis	S. aureus, Streptococci
Congenital heart disease	Streptococci, Haemophilus spp.
Neutropenia	Aerobic gram-negative bacilli, *Aspergillus* spp., *Mucorales, Candida* spp., *Scedosporium* spp.
Transplantation	Aspergillus spp., Candida spp., Mucorales, Scedosporium spp., Enterobacteriaceae, Nocardia spp., Toxoplasma gondii, Mycobacterium tuberculosis
Human immunodeficiency virus infection	T. gondii, Nocardia spp., Mycobacterium spp., Listeria monocytogenes,

Mixed *streptococci* (aerobic, anaerobic, and microaerophilic) are the most common causative agents (60-70%) detected in culture in bacterial brain abscesses. These *streptococci* are present in the oral cavity, the appendix, and the female genital tract and are prone to abscess formation. Group A *streptococci* rarely cause brain abscesses. Advances in culture identification methods and taking effective anaerobic cultures have enabled the detection of causative agents such as *Bacteroides*, the responsible microorganism in 20-40% of brain abscesses. *Enterobacteriaceae* can be isolated at a rate of 25-33%, and S*taphylococcus aureus* can be isolated at a rate of 10-15% as causative agents, especially post-traumatically, after neurosurgical operations, in endocarditis or bacteremic patients. Despite the low detection rates of *Haemophilus influenzae*, *Streptococcus pneumoniae*, and *Listeria monocytogenes* in brain abscesses, they may be causative agents in brain abscesses developing as a complication of meningitis. Abscesses caused by fungi, especially C*andida*, have gradually increased due to the use of broad-spectrum antibiotics and immunosuppression (Fennely, 2013). Upon reviewing the literature, candidal abscesses are usually detected in autopsies. Comorbid conditions associated with candidal abscesses include antibiotic use, previous surgery, malignancy, stem cell or solid organ transplantation, previous use of corticosteroids, central venous catheter (CVC) insertion, and burns (Andrea, 2013). *Aspergillus* spp., *Mucormycosis, Scedosporium* spp., *Cryptococcus neoformans, Coccidioides* spp., *Histoplasma capsulatum* and *Blastomyces dermatitidis* are other fungal causative agents that can cause brain abscesses, particularly in immunosuppressed patients. Toxoplasmosis is the most common protozoal cause of brain abscesses. Their frequency has increased considerably with HIV infections. Nowadays, effective antiretroviral therapy and prophylactic applications have significantly reduced their incidence. Although brain abscesses progress with various clinical findings, intracranial mass, and encephalitis are their most common forms.

The clinical presentation of brain abscesses can range from mild to fulminant. There are usually short-term symptoms lasting for less than two weeks. The virulence of the microorganism and the size of the lesion occupying space in the brain play a role in the development of clinical findings (Bennett, 2015; Bokhari and Mesfin, 2022). Headache, altered state of consciousness, nausea and/or vomiting, and high fever are the most common symptoms. Focal neurological deficits may develop over time. Epileptic seizures, which can be observed in 25-34% of patients, may be a complaint at the first presentation. The sudden worsening headache and subsequent meningismus symptoms may be indicative of abscess rupture. Fever, headache, and focal neurological deficit, known as the classical triad, can be detected in less than 50% of patients. Moreover, the findings may be subtle in immunosuppressed patients. Abscess localization is a determinant in the developing clinical picture. Clinically, ataxia, nystagmus, and vomiting can be observed in cerebellar abscesses; lethargy, inattention, deterioration in mental status, hemiparesis, and motor speech disorder can be observed in frontal lobe abscesses, and a visual field defect can be observed in an abscess in the temporal lobe.

When evaluating patients with suspected brain abscesses, routine tests, such as complete blood count, erythrocyte sedimentation rate, and serum C-reactive protein, and serological tests (e.g., Toxoplasma), when necessary, should be planned, and blood cultures should be taken before starting antibiotics. It is a clinical pathology requiring multidisciplinary management, and infectious diseases require evaluation by a team consisting of neuroradiologists and neurosurgeons. Suspicious patients must be imaged with contrast-enhanced CT or MRI. Radiological findings may vary according to the stage. Early cerebritis is detected as non-enhancing or patchy contrast-enhanced hypodense areas, whereas the lesion becomes more prominent over time. The characteristic CT appearance of brain abscess is a circular hypodense center surrounded by a variable degree of hypodense cerebral edema after contrast medium. Progressively diminishing edema and mass effect are observed on serial CT scans in patients with late abscesses. Magnetic resonance imaging (MRI) is more sensitive for early cerebritis and satellite lesions and predicts lesion necrosis and extent. It provides a greater contrast between cerebral edema and the brain and allows the detection of the spread of inflammation to the ventricles and subarachnoid space. Performing stereotactic CT-guided aspiration, if possible, facilitates diagnosis, provides microbiological sampling, and guides antimicrobial therapy in patients.

Considering the presence of predisposing causes in patients with brain abscesses, the recommended standard antimicrobial regimens should be started empirically. The treatment must be modified according to the causative agent if the causative agent has been isolated. A surgical approach is usually required in addition to medical treatment. Nevertheless, antimicrobial therapy alone may be considered in some groups of patients, including deep localization, small abscesses, multiple abscesses, or the presence of conditions increasing the risk of surgery. The combination of third-generation cephalosporin (ceftriaxone, cefotaxime) and metronidazole is the first-choice treatment regimen to be preferred in patients with brain abscesses, especially predisposing otitis media, sinusitis mastoiditis. A combination of third- or fourth-generation cephalosporin (cefepime) and vancomycin can be used in post-traumatic or post-neurosurgical conditions with the unknown predisposing condition. In immunosuppressed patients, it may be necessary to add antifungal agents or agents such as trimethoprim/sulfamethoxazole according to the suspected causative agents.

The optimal duration of treatment after surgical intervention must be 6-8 weeks. Patients should be followed up by imaging methods, and the necessity of surgery should be re-evaluated in patients in whom the abscess grows after 2 weeks or does not regress with 3-4 weeks of treatment. Shorter treatments of 3-4 weeks may be considered for surgically removed abscesses. Long-term treatment for more than 12 weeks should be planned with close clinical and radiological follow-up in the patient group where surgical treatment is impossible.

Conclusion

In conclusion, epidural abscess, subdural empyema, and brain abscess are CNS infections with a high risk of mortality and morbidity despite all advances in medical and surgical treatments. Clinical suspicion, prompt antimicrobial therapy and surgical intervention, and long-term close follow-up are the most important factors determining patient survival.

References

Abdallah A. (2021). Pediatric Spinal Subdural Abscesses: A Report of Three Consecutive Patients. *Pediatric neurosurgery*, *56*(1), 17–34. https://doi.org/10.1159/000512718.

Akhondi, H., & Baker, M. B. (2022). Epidural Abscess. In *StatPearls*. StatPearls Publishing. NBK535450.

Artenstein, A. W., Friderici, J., Holers, A., Lewis, D., Fitzgerald, J., & Visintainer, P. (2016). Spinal Epidural Abscess in Adults: A 10-Year Clinical Experience at a Tertiary Care Academic Medical Center. *Open forum infectious diseases*, *3*(4), ofw191. https://doi.org/10.1093/ofid/ofw191.

Bennett, J. E., Dolin, R., Blaser, M. J. (Eds.) (2015). Mandell, Douglas, and Bennett's principles and practice of infectious diseases. In Tunkel. A.R. *Subdural Empyema, Epidural Abscess, and Suppurative Intracranial Thrombophlebitis.* (8th edition, 1176-1185) Elsevier. https://doi.org/10.1016/C2012-1-00075-6.

Bennett. J. E., Dolin, R., Blaser. M. J. (Eds.) (2015). Mandell, Douglas, and Bennett's principles and practice of infectious diseases. (Eighth edition). In Tunkel. A.R. *Brain abscess.* (1114-1176) Elsevier. https://doi.org/10.1016/C2012-1-00075-6.

Bokhari, M. R., & Mesfin, F. B. (2022). Brain Abscess. In *Stat Pearls*. StatPearls Publishing.NBK441841.

Carter, J. E., Laurini, J. A., Evans, T. N., &Estrada, B. (2008). Neonatal Candida parapsilosis meningitis and empyem are lated to epidural migration of a central venous catheter. *Clinical neurology and neurosurgery*, *110*(6), 614–618. https://doi.org/10.1016/j.clineuro.2008.03.012.

Davis, D. P., Wold, R. M., Patel, R. J., Tran, A. J., Tokhi, R. N., Chan, T. C., & Vilke, G. M. (2004). The clinical presentation and impact of diagnostic delays on emergency department patients with spinal epidural abscess. *The Journal of emergency medicine*, *26*(3), 285–291. https://doi.org/10.1016/j.jemermed.2003.11.013.

Fennelly, A. M., Slenker, A. K., Murphy, L. C., Moussouttas, M., & DeSimone, J. A. (2013). Candida cerebral abscesses: a case report and review of the literature. *Medical mycology*, *51*(7), 779–784. https://doi.org/10.3109/13693786.2013.789566.

Fernández-de Thomas, R. J., & De Jesus, O. (2023). Subdural Empyema. In *Stat Pearls*. Stat Pearls Publishing. NBK557829.

Hunter, S., Cussen, R., & Baker, J. F. (2021). Predictors of Failure for Nonoperative Management of Spinal Epidural Abscess. *Global spine journal*, *11*(1), 6–12. https://doi.org/10.1177/2192568219887915.

Kapmaz, M., Gülşen, I., Kış, N., Başaran, S., Oksüz, L., & Gürler, N. (2014). A Highly Rare Cause of Lumbar Spondylodiscitis with Epidural Abscess: Actinomyces israelii. *Case reports in infectious diseases*, *2014*, 469075. https://doi.org/10.1155/2014/469075.

Lu, H. F., Yue, C. T., & Kung, W. M. (2022). *Salmonella* Group D1 Subdural Empyema Mimicking Subdural Hematoma: A Case Report. *Infection and drug resistance*, *15*, 6357–6363. https://doi.org/10.2147/IDR.S388101.

Martínez de Pinillos Sánchez, M. V., Amat Serna, T., & Gordillo Resina, M. M. (2022). Nocardia abscess us epidural abscess. *Medicina intensiva*, *46*(10), 598–600. https://doi.org/10.1016/j.medine.2022.06.016.

Reihsaus, E., Waldbaur, H., &Seeling, W. (2000). Spinal epidural abscess: a meta-analysis of 915 patients. *Neurosurgical review*, *23*(4), 175–205. https://doi.org/10.1007/pl00011954.

Ren, J., Yap, J., & Donaldson, J., (2023). *Spinal epidural abscess*. Reference article, Radiopaedia.org (Accessed on 21 Mar 2023) https://doi.org/10.53347/rID-28899.

Sanford (2023). *The Sanford guide to antimicrobial therapy*. Dallas, TX: Antimicrobial Therapy, Inc.

Schwab, J. H., &Shah, A. A. (2020). Spinal Epidural Abscess: Diagnosis, Management, and Outcomes. *The Journal of the American Academy of Orthopaedic Surgeons*, *28*(21), e929–e938. https://doi.org/10.5435/JAAOS-D-19-00685.

Shah, A. A., Ogink, P. T., Nelson, S. B., Harris, M. B., & Schwab, J. H. (2018). Nonoperative Management of Spinal Epidural Abscess: Development of a Predictive Algorithm for Failure. *The Journal of bone and joint surgery. American volume*, *100* (7), 546–555. https://doi.org/10.2106/JBJS.17.00629.

Silverberg, A. L., & Di Nubile, M. J. (1985). Subdural empyema and cranial epidural abscess. *The Medical clinics of North America*, *69*(2), 361–374. https://doi.org/10.1016/s0025-7125(16)31048-3.

So, G., Haraguchi, W., & Kinoshita, N. (2018). *No shinkei geka. Neurological surgery*, *46*(7), 623–628. https://doi.org/10.11477/mf.1436203780.

Sobottke, R., Röllinghoff, M., Zarghooni, K., Zarghooni, K., Schlüter-Brust, K., Delank, K. S., Seifert, H., Zweig, T., & Eysel, P. (2010). Spondylodiscitis in the elderly patient: clinical mid-term results and quality of life. *Archives of orthopaedic and trauma surgery*, *130*(9), 1083–1091. https://doi.org/10.1007/s00402-009-0972-z.

Wu, T. J., Chiu, N. C., & Huang, F. Y. (2008). Subdural empyema in children--20-year experience in a medical center. *Journal of microbiology, immunology, and infection = Wei mian yu gan ran za zhi*, *41*(1), 62–67.

Chapter 9

Rabies and the Central Nervous System

Özgen Gönenç Çekiç*, MD
Department of Emergency Medicine, Faculty of Medicine, University of Health Science, Trabzon, Turkiye

Abstract

Rabies is a neglected zoonotic disease that affects the central nervous system. Rabies is usually transmitted to humans by animal bites, and dogs are the most important vector worldwide. It is estimated that canine rabies causes approximately 59,000 deaths annually. There are encephalitic and paralytic forms of the disease. Neuroimaging is non-specific. Confirmatory diagnostic laboratory tests for rabies include the detection of neutralizing anti-rabies virus antibodies in serum or cerebrospinal fluid and rabies virus antigen or RNA in tissues or fluids. Rabies is virtually always fatal after the clinical disease develops, and there have been only a few survivors.

Keywords: rabies, viral encephalitis, central nervous system

Introduction

Rabies is a terrifying public health problem worldwide that has affected humans over centuries. As revealed by the initial records found in Mesopotamia, this zoonosis has been present throughout recorded history. The term Rabies originates from the Latin word *rabere*, which means a state of madness (Baer, 1994).

---

* Corresponding Author's Email: ozgen_gonencc@hotmail.com.

In: Central Nervous System Infections
Editor: Mustafa Usanmaz
ISBN: 979-8-89113-660-1

Rabies is a fatal zoonotic infection with rabies virus (RABV) transmission by animal bites that produces encephalitis in humans and other mammals. RABV belongs to the Rhabdoviridae family and the genus Lyssavirus; it is characterized as a negative strand RNA virus (Albertini et al., 2011). Lyssaviruses are enveloped single-stranded RNA viruses that have a bullet-shaped morphology (Natesan et al., 2023). The genus Lyssavirus includes 17 recognized species, with the most well-known being rabies virus (serotype 1), which is responsible for the majority of human deaths from lyssavirus infections (Rupprecht et al., 1995; Walker et al., 2018).

Epidemiology

Rabies occurs worldwide and on all continents except Antarctica. Determining the exact incidence of rabies is challenging due to factors such as poor enforcement of existing legislation, limited access to approved diagnostic tests and reagents, and the lower socioeconomic status of certain regions, particularly in Asia and Africa (Taylor et al., 2017). However, the mortality from rabies is notably underestimated in numerous regions around the world. Annually, an estimated 59,000 deaths are caused by canine rabies, particularly in developing countries. The reported deaths likely underestimate the global incidence of the disease, which is believed to result in up to 159,000 deaths annually (Hampson et al., 2015). In countries where rabies is endemic, a disproportionate number of those affected are children (Baker et al., 2022). In developed countries, the incidence of rabies is much lower due to widespread vaccination of domestic animals and effective post-exposure prophylaxis for humans (Riccardi et al., 2021).

The disease affects all warm-blooded animals, including humans. The primary route of viral transmission involves the introduction of virus-containing saliva into muscle tissue or other peripheral tissues, often occurring as a consequence of animal bites. Canines serve as the primary reservoir for rabies viruses, with dog bites contributing to over 99% of human occurences (Fooks et al., 2017). In Asian countries, dogs are the major animal reservoirs for rabies transmission, whereas in America, Africa, and Eurasia, transmission facilitated by bats and other animals presents a significant risk (Ma et al., 2018; Sudarshan et al., 2007). In addition to the primary routes of transmission, there are other potential ways in which rabies can be transmitted. Among these instances are cases of organ transplantation from donors with undiagnosed rabies, which have led to fatal outcomes among transplant recipients (Chen et al., 2017; Srinivasan et al., 2005). Moreover, while infrequent, infection through the aerosol route has also been documented (Johnson et al., 2006).

Main Body

Pathogenesis

RABV infects muscle cells after inoculation and replicates therein at a low rate before nervous system infection occurs. The initial molecular targets recognized for the rabies virus were nicotinic acetylcholine receptors (Lentz et al., 1983). The list of targets has been expanded to include the metabotropic glutamate receptor subtype 2, the p75 neurotophin receptor, the neural cell adhesion molecule, and the integrin ß, all of which facilitate viral entry into the cell (Lafon, 2005; Lian et al., 2022; Wang et al., 2018). The timely administration of rabies immune globulin (RIG) and active immunization can effectively halt the virus from advancing into the nervous system, preventing its spread. RABV is unable to survive in environments with a pH below 3 or above 11. Furthermore, sunlight, ultraviolet light, and specific chemicals such as formalin and detergents, lead to its inactivation.

After an incubation period that usually lasts for weeks or months, RABV enters the peripheral nervous system (PNS) through motor endplates at the neuromuscular junction. Once the virus has entered the peripheral nerves, current therapeutic techniques are unlikely to effectively prevent subsequent replication and spread. The virus quickly progresses from neuron to neuron towards the central nervous system (CNS) at about 50-100 mm per day (Warrell & Warrell, 2004). From there, the virus spreads within the peripheral nerves using microtubule dependent retrograde fast axonal transport, eventually reaching the spinal cord or brainstem, depending on the site of inoculation (Ugolini, 2011). Subsequently, the virus spreads throughout the CNS by following neuroanatomical connections (Scott & Nel, 2021). After CNS infection, RABV can spread to peripheral, non-neuronal organs (e.g., the adrenal gland, heart, skin, and salivary gland) anterograde transport and can be detected at these sites after the onset of clinical symptoms (Potratz et al., 2020). On the contrary, centrifugal spread occurs at a slower rate, with passive diffusion likely facilitating the process instead of active transport (Ugolini, 2011).

Histopathology

The neuropathology of rabies is characterized by mild inflammatory changes, edema, and the presence of intracytoplasmic eosinophilic inclusion bodies known as Negri bodies. Negri bodies, the pathognomonic microscobic finding, are most commonly found in the pyramidal neurons of the hippocampus and in cerebellar Purkinje cells (Jackson et al., 2001). Additionally, more irregularly demarcated inclusions, called Lyssa bodies, can also be observed. Demonstration of viral nucleocapsid antigens by immunohistochemistry or immunofluorescence is necessary to confirm the diagnosis of rabies encephalitis (Stein et al., 2010).

Clinical Manifestations

Human Rabies

As with other infectious diseases, infection and disease development are not guaranteed by exposure alone. The risk of rabies transmission after exposure is influenced by several factors, including the type and anatomical location of the exposure (Fishbein & Robinson, 1993). An animal bite that involves significant salivary contamination, such as direct contact with exposed skin, poses a higher risk of rabies transmission compared to a bite that occurs through thick clothing, which can help remove saliva from the animal's teeth. Also, bites targeted at the face have a higher probability of resulting in disease compared to bites directed at the extremities (Whitehouse et al., 2022). Additionally, host susceptibility to infection and the chances of developing the disease can be influenced by factors such as the size of the viral inoculum, the viral variant, the degree of innervation at the bite site, the host's immune response, and genetic factors (Hemachudha et al., 2013).

Incubation Period

The incubation period of rabies after exposure can vary significantly, ranging from a few days to several years. However, the majority of patients typically develop symptoms within the initial 90 days after exposure. In solid organ transplant recipients, most patients manifest the onset of symptoms within 6 weeks after transplantation (Zhou et al., 2016). Additionally, an exceptional case of a patient who developed the illness 18 months after kidney transplantation has been reported (Vora et al., 2013).

Prodromal Symptoms

The prodromal stage of rabies typically lasts for two to ten days and is characterized by non-specific symptoms such as fever, malaise, headache, fatigue, anorexia, myalgia, nausea, and vomiting. It is important to note that these symptoms are non-specific and can occur in many other viral infections. The first specific clinical symptom of rabies is neuropatic pain or paresthesia at the site of the bite. Pain is a result of virus replication in the dorsal root ganglia and inflammation provoked by cellular immunity (Mitrabhakdi et al., 2005). Cases of bat exposure were more likely to exhibit symptoms localized to the wound compared to dog rabies exposures (Udow et al., 2013). Furthermore, during the prodromal stage and the course of rabies, percussion myoedema (formation of a mound in the muscle upon percussion) can be noted (Hemachudha et al., 1987).

Encephalitic Rabies

Human RABV infection can manifest in two forms, namely encephalitic (furious or classical) and paralytic (dumb) rabies, both starting with nonspecific prodromal symptoms, as mentioned above. The encephalitic manifestation of rabies is predominant, occurring in around 80% of patients, and is characterized by fever, hydrophobia, aerophobia, hyperactivity, and agitation (Ugolini & Hemachudha, 2018). Hydrophobia is the most characteristic symptom of encephalitic rabies and represents an exaggerated irritant reflex of the respiratory tract, possibly arising from infection involving brainstem neurons that inhibit inspiratory motor neurons (Warrell et al., 1976).

Aerophobia, known as fear of drafts or fresh air, is also a pathognomonic disease of rabies. Hydrophobia and aerophobia occur only in humans with rabies but are neither sufficiently sensitive nor specific (Willoughby, 2015). Autonomic dysfunction is also observed, including pupillary dilation, hypersalivation, and sweating (Jackson, 2016). The effects of rabies on the heart, such as myocarditis and cardiac arrhythmias have been reported in several cases (Alexander et al., 2021).

Patients may demonstrate the presence of hallucinations and delirium and, as the disease progresses, seizures may manifest. Other features include meningism, polyuria due to diabetes insipidus, pharyngeal spasms, and hypersexuality (Warrell et al., 2017). Despite maximum supportive care, rabies virtually always results in a fatal outcome within 14 days after initial symptoms (Jackson, 2016). Death is typically caused by respiratory failure and vascular collapse in patients.

Paralytic Rabies

In paralytic form, which is less than 20% of patients with rabies, it is characterized by progressive lower motor neuron weakness mimicking acute inflammatory polyneuropathy (Guillain-Barre syndrome) or a symmetrical quadriparesis (Jackson, 2018; Sheikh et al., 2005). Ascending paralysis, usually most prominent in the bitten limb, progresses rapidly to quadriparesis. Other symptoms such as headache, fever, sensory symptoms, and sphincter dysfunction can be found in patients, and in the later course, paralysis of the deglutition and respiration muscles can occur, ultimately leading to death. Survival in patients with paralytic rabies is longer than in the encephalitic form, likely due to the later involvement of vital brainstem areas (Udow et al., 2013).

Diagnosis

Rabies is an acute, progressive encephalitis. Without a clear-cut rabid bite history, the clinical diagnosis of rabies can be difficult and requires a high index of suspicion (Venkatesan et al., 2013). Therefore, patients, with or without a history of exposure, presenting with symptoms of either agitated or paralytic encephalitic illness should be assessed for a possible diagnosis of rabies. Antemortem rabies diagnosis requires multiple specimens (e.g., serum, skin, saliva, and cerebrospinal fluid (CSF)) and diverse testing methods due to the limited sensitivity of individual tests (Dacheux et al., 2010).

The present diagnostic tools are inadequate for detecting rabies infection prior to the initiation of clinical disease. One or more of the following laboratory criteria should be used to confirm a clinical case, according to the World Health Organization (WHO): the presence of viral antigens in samples (e.g., skin, brain tissue), the isolation of the virus from samples in laboratory animals or in cell culture, the presence of viral-specific antibodies in the serum or CSF of an unvaccinated person, and/or the presence of viral nucleic acids in samples (e.g., skin, saliva,brain tissue, concentrated urine) (Table 1) (Organization, 2018).

Viral antigens in skin biopsy samples or hair follicles from patients with clinical rabies can be detected with a fluorescent antibody test (FAT). FAT is an efficient, sensitive, and specific diagnostic method utilized in both animals and humans to identify rabies. It is widely recognized as the gold standard for diagnosis (Robardet et al., 2011). Typically, skin samples are extracted from the nuchal region of the neck, where hair follicles contain peripheral nerves (Bryceson et al., 1975).

Table 1. Standard diagnostic tests for rabies (Organization, 2018)

	Antigen detection		RNA detection		Virus isolation		Antibody detection	
Time of test	Sample	Test	Sample	Test	Sample	Test	Sample	Test
Human (ante-mortem)[1]	Skin/hair follicles	FAT	Skin/hair follicles Saliva Tears CSF	RT-PCR[2]	Saliva Tears CSF	RTCIT	Serum CSF	RFFIT FAVN-test IFA ELISA
Human (post-mortem	Brain Skin/hair follicles	FAT DRIT IHC	Brain Skin/hair follicles	RT-PCR	Brain	RTCIT MI	-	-

Abbreviations: CSF, cerebrospinal fluid; DRIT, direct rapid immunohistochemical test; ELISA, enzyme-linked immunosorbent assay; FAT, direct fluorescent antibody test; FAVN, fluorescent antibody virus neutralization; IFA, indirect immunofluorescence; IHC, immunohistochemistry in formalin-fixed samples; MI, Mouse inoculation test; RTCIT, rabies cell culture inoculation test; RT-PCR, reverse transcriptasepolymerase chain reaction; RFFIT, rapid fluorescent focus inhibition test.

[1] Positive results in ante-mortem samples are diagnostic, but negative results do not rule out rabies.

[2] RT-PCR may be in the conventional or real-time format.

Another diagnostic method in patients suspected of rabies is RNA detection via reverse transcriptase polymerase chain reaction (RT-PCR) in biopsy samples and saliva (Faye et al., 2017). The highest sensitivity is seen with a skin biopsy or saliva, and optimal diagnostic sensitivity is achieved by obtaining a minimum of three saliva samples (Dacheux et al., 2008). Considering the pathogenesis of rabies, antibodies specific for the rabies virus might be detectable in serum and CSF only during the advanced phase of infection. The gold standard tests recommended by WHO to detect neutralizing antibodies in serum and CSF from individuals previously vaccinated and/or subjects suspected of RABV infection are currently the rapid fluorescent focus inhibition test (RFFIT) and the fluorescent antibody virus neutralization test (FAVN) (Ciconello et al., 2022). Additionally, detection of antibodies and routine screening to assess the development of an immune response after pre- or post-exposure vaccination can be facilitated through the use of enzyme-linked immunosorbent assay (ELISA) (Feyssaguet et al., 2007; Rodriguez et al., 2021).

Radiological findings in rabies encephalitis are generally non-specific and can vary widely depending on the stage of the disease and the severity of inflammation in the CNS. Computed tomography scans of the brain may reveal non-specific hypodens lesions or areas, which can suggest inflammation or necrosis. Magnetic resonance (MR) images show T2 hyperintense signal changes in the hippocampus, brainstem, thalamus, limbic cortex, or hypothalamus (Ramli & Bae, 2023). Depending on the stage of the disease, spinal cord involvement in MR can be noted, particularly in paralytic rabies (Kalita et al., 2014). Gray matter involvement is typically seen in rabies encephalitis, whereas white matter is primarily affected in acute disseminated encephalomyelitis (ADEM) (Santhoshkumar et al., 2012).

Differential Diagnosis

The prodromal phase can be confused with various disorders, such as nonspesific viral illness, mononucleosis, bacteremia, or meningitis. In patients presenting with symptoms of encephalitic rabies, it is important to rule out other viral encephalitis infections such as the herpes simplex virus and the West Nile virus. Herpes simplex encephalitis, which is the most common form of sporadically occurring fatal encephalitis in humans, can mimic rabies (Feige et al., 2021). Other differential diagnostic considerations include tetanus, cerebral malaria, and strychnine poisoning (Mudiyanselage et al., 2016). The paralytic form may resemble Guillain-Barre syndrome, West Nile virus infection, and polimyelitis (Mateen & Black, 2013; Sheikh et al., 2005).

Treatment

Rabies is widely recognized as a fatal disease, with only a few documented cases of survival. There is no viable curative treatment for rabies once clinical signs have become evident. The majority of survivors thus far have experienced severe neurological complications and have received one or more doses of the rabies vaccine before the onset of clinical rabies (Jackson, 2016). In the management of patients with confirmed or suspected rabies, two management approaches can be considered: a palliative approach or an aggressive approach.

Palliative Treatment

The palliative approach can be implemented either in a hospital setting or in the comfort of the patient's home. This approach involves providing sedation, adequate hydration, and care in a suitable medical facility in a quiet room, accompanied by appropriate physical and emotional support (Tarantola et al.,

2016). Dehydration can be prevented by administering intravenous (IV) or other possible parenteral routes for hydration (Thomas & Barclay, 2015). Sedation and muscle relaxation can be achieved effectively through the administration of benzodiazepins such as diazepam. Diazepam can be administered IV at a dose of 10 mg for 3-5 minutes, with repeat doses given every 1-4 hours. Alternatively, it can be administered intrarectally at a dose of 10 mg every 1-4 hours. Additionally, for the treatment of fever, paracetamol can be used at a dose of 1 g every 4-6 hours (Warrell et al., 2017). Anticholinergic agents such as scopolamine can be utilized to manage excessive salivation.

Aggressive Treatment

Supportive care in a critical care unit is essential for an aggressive approach. Experimental agressive protocols, such as the Milwaukee protocol, have been used in patients with rabies (Willoughby et al., 2005). This protocol includes inducing a therapeutic coma using benzodiazepines and phenobarbital, as well as administering ketamine and antiviral therapy with ribavirin and amantadine. None of these treatments can be supported in cases of rabies or other types of acute viral encephalitis (Zeiler & Jackson, 2016). Antiviral agents, including ribavirin, amantadine, interferon-α, and favipiravir, are used in treatment, although there is a lack of evidence supporting their efficacy in humans (Appolinario & Jackson, 2015; Yamada et al., 2016).

When considering the implementation of a potential aggresive treatment approach for a patient with rabies, it is important to acknowledge that rabies is almost always fatal, and there is no reliable means to predict which patients are likely to recover.

Conclusion

For centuries, rabies has been a terrifying and deadly zoonotic disease for humankind. Although the eradication of rabies is currently not considered feasible, the disease persists in the wild as an affliction that affects the central nervous system. While medical progress has led to advancements in rabies diagnosis, these developments have not been mirrored in the field of treatment.

References

Albertini, A. A., Ruigrok, R. W., & Blondel, D. (2011). Rabies virus transcription and replication. *Adv Virus Res*, *79*, 1-22. https://doi.org/10.1016/B978-0-12-387040-7.00001-9.

Alexander, B., Lopez-Lopez, J. P., Saldarriaga, C., Ponte-Negretti, C. I., Lopez-Santi, R., Perez, G. E., Del Sueldo, M., Lanas, F., Liblik, K., & Baranchuk, A. (2021). Rabies and the Heart. *Cardiol Res*, *12*(2), 53-59. https://doi.org/10.14740/cr1216.

Appolinario, C. M., & Jackson, A. C. (2015). Antiviral therapy for human rabies. *Antivir Ther*, *20*(1), 1-10. https://doi.org/10.3851/IMP2851.

Baer, G. M. (1994). Rabies--an historical perspective. *Infect Agents Dis*, *3*(4), 168-180. https://www.ncbi.nlm.nih.gov/pubmed/7827785.

Baker, H. J., Martin, D. R., Gross, A. L., Chamorro, M. F., Naskou, M. C., Johnson, A. K., Brock, K. V., Van Kampen, K. R., & Willoughby, R. E. (2022). Rabies: who should care? *J Am Vet Med Assoc*, *261*(4), 592-596. https://doi.org/10.2460/javma.22.09.0420.

Bryceson, A. D., Greenwood, B. M., Warrell, D. A., Davidson, N. M., Pope, H. M., Lawrie, J. H., Barnes, J., Bailie, W. E., & Wilcox, G. E. (1975). Demonstration during life of rabies antigen in humans. *J Infect Dis*, *131*(1), 71-74. https://doi.org/10.1093/infdis/131.1.71.

Chen, S., Zhang, H., Luo, M., Chen, J., Yao, D., Chen, F., Liu, R, & Chen, T. (2017). Rabies Virus Transmission in Solid Organ Transplantation, China, 2015-2016. *Emerg Infect Dis*, *23*(9), 1600-1602. https://doi.org/10.3201/eid2309.161704.

Ciconello, F. N., Katz, I. S. S., Fernandes, E. R., Guedes, F., & Silva, S. R. (2022). A comparative review of serological assays for the detection of rabies virus-specific antibodies. *Acta Trop*, *226*, 106254. https://doi.org/10.1016/j.actatropica.2021.106254.

Dacheux, L., Reynes, J. M., Buchy, P., Sivuth, O., Diop, B. M., Rousset, D., Rathat, C., Jolly, N., Dufourcq, J. B., Nareth, C., Diop, S., Iehlé, C., Rajerison, R., Sadorge, C., & Bourhy, H. (2008). A reliable diagnosis of human rabies based on analysis of skin biopsy specimens. *Clin Infect Dis*, *47*(11), 1410-1417. https://doi.org/10.1086/592969.

Dacheux, L., Wacharapluesadee, S., Hemachudha, T., Meslin, F. X., Buchy, P., Reynes, J. M., & Bourhy, H. (2010). More accurate insight into the incidence of human rabies in developing countries through validated laboratory techniques. *PLoS Negl Trop Dis*, *4*(11), e765. https://doi.org/10.1371/journal.pntd.0000765.

Faye, M., Dacheux, L., Weidmann, M., Diop, S. A., Loucoubar, C., Bourhy, H., Sall, H., & Faye, O. (2017). Development and validation of sensitive real-time RT-PCR assay for broad detection of rabies virus. *J Virol Methods*, *243*, 120-130. https://doi.org/10.1016/j.jviromet.2016.12.019.

Feige, L., Zaeck, L. M., Sehl-Ewert, J., Finke, S., & Bourhy, H. (2021). Innate Immune Signaling and Role of Glial Cells in Herpes Simplex Virus- and Rabies Virus-Induced Encephalitis. *Viruses*, *13*(12). https://doi.org/10.3390/v13122364.

Feyssaguet, M., Dacheux, L., Audry, L., Compoint, A., Morize, J. L., Blanchard, I., & Bourhy, H. (2007). Multicenter comparative study of a new ELISA, PLATELIA

RABIES II, for the detection and titration of anti-rabies glycoprotein antibodies and comparison with the rapid fluorescent focus inhibition test (RFFIT) on human samples from vaccinated and non-vaccinated people. *Vaccine*, *25*(12), 2244-2251. https://doi.org/10.1016/j.vaccine.2006.12.012.

Fishbein, D. B., & Robinson, L. E. (1993). Rabies. *N Engl J Med*, *329*(22), 1632-1638. https://doi.org/10.1056/NEJM199311253292208.

Fooks, A. R., Cliquet, F., Finke, S., Freuling, C., Hemachudha, T., Mani, R. S., Müller T, Nadin-Davis S, Picard-Meyer E, Wilde H, & Banyard, A. C. (2017). Rabies. *Nat Rev Dis Primers*, *3*, 17091. https://doi.org/10.1038/nrdp.2017.91.

Hampson, K., Coudeville, L., Lembo, T., Sambo, M., Kieffer, A., Attlan, M., Barrat, J., Blanton, J. D., Briggs, D. J., Cleaveland, S., Costa, P., Freuling, C. M., Hiby, E., Knopf, L., Leanes, F., Meslin, F. X., Metlin, A., Miranda, M. E., Müller, T., Nel, L. H., Recuenco, S., Rupprecht, C. E., Schumacher, C., Taylor, L., Vigilato, M. A., Zinsstag, J., Dushoff, J. & Global Alliance for Rabies Control Partners for Rabies, P. (2015). Estimating the global burden of endemic canine rabies. *PLoS Negl Trop Dis*, *9*(4), e0003709. https://doi.org/10.1371/journal.pntd.0003709.

Hemachudha, T., Phanthumchinda, K., Phanuphak, P., & Manutsathit, S. (1987). Myoedema as a clinical sign in paralytic rabies. *Lancet*, *1*(8543), 1210. https://doi.org/10.1016/s0140-6736(87)92186-6.

Hemachudha, T., Ugolini, G., Wacharapluesadee, S., Sungkarat, W., Shuangshoti, S., & Laothamatas, J. (2013). Human rabies: neuropathogenesis, diagnosis, and management. *Lancet Neurol*, *12*(5), 498-513. https://doi.org/10.1016/S1474-4422(13) 70038-3.

Jackson, A. C. (2016). Human Rabies: a 2016 Update. *Curr Infect Dis Rep*, *18*(11), 38. https://doi.org/10.1007/s11908-016-0540-y.

Jackson, A. C. (2018). Rabies: a medical perspective. *Rev Sci Tech*, *37*(2), 569-580. https://doi.org/10.20506/rst.37.2.2825 (Rabies: a medical perspective.).

Jackson, A. C., Ye, H., Ridaura-Sanz, C., & Lopez-Corella, E. (2001). Quantitative study of the infection in brain neurons in human rabies. *J Med Virol*, *65*(3), 614-618. https://www.ncbi.nlm.nih.gov/pubmed/11596101.

Johnson, N., Phillpotts, R., & Fooks, A. R. (2006). Airborne transmission of lyssaviruses. *J Med Microbiol*, *55*(Pt 6), 785-790. https://doi.org/10.1099/jmm.0.46370-0.

Kalita, J., Bhoi, S. K., Bastia, J. K., Lashkar, S., Mahadevan, A., & Misra, U. K. (2014). Paralytic rabies: MRI findings and review of literature. *Neurol India*, *62*(6), 662-664. https://doi.org/10.4103/0028-3886.149394.

Lafon, M. (2005). Rabies virus receptors. *J Neurovirol*, *11*(1), 82-87. https://doi.org/10.1080/13550280590900427.

Lentz, T. L., Burrage, T. G., Smith, A. L., & Tignor, G. H. (1983). The acetylcholine receptor as a cellular receptor for rabies virus. *Yale J Biol Med*, *56*(4), 315-322. https://www.ncbi.nlm.nih.gov/pubmed/6367238.

Lian, M., Hueffer, K., & Weltzin, M. M. (2022). Interactions between the rabies virus and nicotinic acetylcholine receptors: A potential role in rabies virus induced behavior modifications. *Heliyon*, *8*(9), e10434. https://doi.org/10.1016/j.heliyon.2022.e10434.

Ma, X., Monroe, B. P., Cleaton, J. M., Orciari, L. A., Li, Y., Kirby, J. D., Chipman, R. B., Petersen, B. W., Wallace, R. M., & Blanton, J. D. (2018). Rabies surveillance in the

United States during 2017. *J Am Vet Med Assoc*, *253*(12), 1555-1568. https://doi.org/10.2460/javma.253.12.1555.

Mateen, F. J., & Black, R. E. (2013). Expansion of acute flaccid paralysis surveillance: beyond poliomyelitis. *Trop Med Int Health*, *18*(11), 1421-1422. https://doi.org/10.1111/tmi.12181.

Mitrabhakdi, E., Shuangshoti, S., Wannakrairot, P., Lewis, R. A., Susuki, K., Laothamatas, J., & Hemachudha, T. (2005). Difference in neuropathogenetic mechanisms in human furious and paralytic rabies. *J Neurol Sci*, *238*(1-2), 3-10. https://doi.org/10.1016/j.jns.2005.05.004.

Mudiyanselage, M. H., Weerasinghe, N. P., Pathirana, K., & Dias, H. (2016). Misdiagnosis of cerebral malaria initially as acute psychotic disorder and later as human rabies: a case report. *BMC Res Notes*, *9*(1), 400. https://doi.org/10.1186/s13104-016-2211-3.

Natesan, K., Isloor, S., Vinayagamurthy, B., Ramakrishnaiah, S., Doddamane, R., & Fooks, A. R. (2023). Developments in Rabies Vaccines: The Path Traversed from Pasteur to the Modern Era of Immunization. *Vaccines (Basel)*, *11*(4). https://doi.org/10.3390/vaccines11040756.

Organization, W. H. (2018). *WHO expert consultation on rabies: third report* (Vol. 1012). World Health Organization.

Potratz, M., Zaeck, L. M., Weigel, C., Klein, A., Freuling, C. M., Muller, T., & Finke, S. (2020). Neuroglia infection by rabies virus after anterograde virus spread in peripheral neurons. *Acta Neuropathol Commun*, *8*(1), 199. https://doi.org/10.1186/s40478-020-01074-6.

Ramli, N. M., & Bae, Y. J. (2023). Structured Imaging Approach for Viral Encephalitis. *Neuroimaging Clin N Am*, *33*(1), 43-56. https://doi.org/10.1016/j.nic.2022.07.002.

Riccardi, N., Giacomelli, A., Antonello, R. M., Gobbi, F., & Angheben, A. (2021). Rabies in Europe: An epidemiological and clinical update. *Eur J Intern Med*, *88*, 15-20. https://doi.org/10.1016/j.ejim.2021.04.010.

Robardet, E., Picard-Meyer, E., Andrieu, S., Servat, A., & Cliquet, F. (2011). International interlaboratory trials on rabies diagnosis: an overview of results and variation in reference diagnosis techniques (fluorescent antibody test, rabies tissue culture infection test, mouse inoculation test) and molecular biology techniques. *J Virol Methods*, *177*(1), 15-25. https://doi.org/10.1016/j.jviromet.2011.06.004.

Rodriguez, M. C., Fontana, D., Garay, E., & Prieto, C. (2021). Detection and quantification of anti-rabies glycoprotein antibodies: current state and perspectives. *Appl Microbiol Biotechnol*, *105*(18), 6547-6557. https://doi.org/10.1007/s00253-021-11515-4.

Rupprecht, C. E., Smith, J. S., Fekadu, M., & Childs, J. E. (1995). The ascension of wildlife rabies: a cause for public health concern or intervention? *Emerg Infect Dis*, *1*(4), 107-114. https://doi.org/10.3201/eid0104.950401.

Santhoshkumar, A., Kalpana, D., & Sowrabha, R. (2012). Rabies encephalomyelitis vs. ADEM: Usefulness of MR imaging in differential diagnosis. *J Pediatr Neurosci*, *7*(2), 133-135. https://doi.org/10.4103/1817-1745.102578.

Scott, T. P., & Nel, L. H. (2021). Lyssaviruses and the Fatal Encephalitic Disease Rabies. *Front Immunol*, *12*, 786953. https://doi.org/10.3389/fimmu.2021.786953.

Sheikh, K. A., Ramos-Alvarez, M., Jackson, A. C., Li, C. Y., Asbury, A. K., & Griffin, J. W. (2005). Overlap of pathology in paralytic rabies and axonal Guillain-Barre syndrome. *Ann Neurol*, *57*(5), 768-772. https://doi.org/10.1002/ana.20482.

Srinivasan, A., Burton, E. C., Kuehnert, M. J., Rupprecht, C., Sutker, W. L., Ksiazek, T. G., . Paddock, C. D., Guarner, J., Shieh, W. J., Goldsmith, C., Hanlon, C. A., Zoretic, J., Fischbach, B., Niezgoda, M., El-Feky, W. H., Orciari, L., Sanchez, E. Q., Likos, A., Klintmalm, G. B., Cardo, D., LeDuc, J., Chamberland, M. E., Jernigan, D. B., Zaki, S. R. & Rabies in Transplant Recipients Investigation, T. (2005). Transmission of rabies virus from an organ donor to four transplant recipients. *N Engl J Med*, *352*(11), 1103-1111. https://doi.org/10.1056/NEJMoa043018.

Stein, L. T., Rech, R. R., Harrison, L., & Brown, C. C. (2010). Immunohistochemical study of rabies virus within the central nervous system of domestic and wildlife species. *Vet Pathol*, *47*(4), 630-633. https://doi.org/10.1177/0300985810370013.

Sudarshan, M. K., Madhusudana, S. N., Mahendra, B. J., Rao, N. S., Ashwath Narayana, D. H., Abdul Rahman, S., Meslin, F., Lobo, D., Ravikumar, K., & Gangaboraiah. (2007). Assessing the burden of human rabies in India: results of a national multi-center epidemiological survey. *Int J Infect Dis*, *11*(1), 29-35. https://doi.org/10.1016/j.ijid.2005.10.007.

Tarantola, A., Crabol, Y., Mahendra, B. J., In, S., Barennes, H., Bourhy, H., Peng Y, Ly S, & Buchy, P. (2016). Caring for patients with rabies in developing countries - the neglected importance of palliative care. *Trop Med Int Health*, *21*(4), 564-567. https://doi.org/10.1111/tmi.12670.

Taylor, L. H., Hampson, K., Fahrion, A., Abela-Ridder, B., & Nel, L. H. (2017). Difficulties in estimating the human burden of canine rabies. *Acta Trop*, *165*, 133-140. https://doi.org/10.1016/j.actatropica.2015.12.007.

Thomas, T., & Barclay, S. (2015). Continuous subcutaneous infusion in palliative care: a review of current practice. *Int J Palliat Nurs*, *21*(2), 60, 62-64. https://doi.org/10.12968/ijpn.2015.21.2.60.

Udow, S. J., Marrie, R. A., & Jackson, A. C. (2013). Clinical features of dog- and bat-acquired rabies in humans. *Clin Infect Dis*, *57*(5), 689-696. https://doi.org/10.1093/cid/cit372.

Ugolini, G. (2011). Rabies virus as a transneuronal tracer of neuronal connections. *Adv Virus Res*, *79*, 165-202. https://doi.org/10.1016/B978-0-12-387040-7.00010-X.

Ugolini, G., & Hemachudha, T. (2018). Rabies: changing prophylaxis and new insights in pathophysiology. *Curr Opin Infect Dis*, *31*(1), 93-101. https://doi.org/10.1097/QCO.0000000000000420.

Venkatesan, A., Tunkel, A. R., Bloch, K. C., Lauring, A. S., Sejvar, J., Bitnun, A., Stahl, J. P., Mailles, A., Drebot, M., Rupprecht, C. E., Yoder, J,. Cope, J. R., Wilson, M. R., Whitley, R. J., Sullivan, J., Granerod, J., Jones, C., Eastwood, K., Ward, K. N., Durrheim, D. N., Solbrig, M. V., Guo-Dong, L., Glaser, C. A., & International Encephalitis, C. (2013). Case definitions, diagnostic algorithms, and priorities in encephalitis: consensus statement of the international encephalitis consortium. *Clin Infect Dis*, *57*(8), 1114-1128. https://doi.org/10.1093/cid/cit458.

Vora, N. M., Basavaraju, S. V., Feldman, K. A., Paddock, C. D., Orciari, L., Gitterman, S., Griese, S., Wallace, R. M., Said, M., Blau, D. M., Selvaggi, G., Velasco-Villa, A.,

Ritter, J., Yager, P., Kresch, A., Niezgoda, M., Blanton, J., Stosor, V., Falta, E. M., Lyon, G. M. 3rd, Zembower, T., Kuzmina, N., Rohatgi, P. K., Recuenco, S., Zaki, S., Damon, I., Franka, R., Kuehnert, M. J., & Transplant-Associated Rabies Virus Transmission Investigation, T. (2013). Raccoon rabies virus variant transmission through solid organ transplantation. *JAMA*, *310*(4), 398-407. https://doi.org/10.1001/jama.2013.7986.

Walker, P. J., Blasdell, K. R., Calisher, C. H., Dietzgen, R. G., Kondo, H., Kurath, G., London, B., Stone D. M., Tesh, R. B., Tordo, N., Vasilakis, N., Whitfield, A. E., & Ictv Report, C. (2018). ICTV Virus Taxonomy Profile: Rhabdoviridae. *J Gen Virol*, *99*(4), 447-448. https://doi.org/10.1099/jgv.0.001020.

Wang, J., Wang, Z., Liu, R., Shuai, L., Wang, X., Luo, J., Wang, C., Chen, W., Wang, X., Ge, J., He, X., Wen, Z., & Bu, Z. (2018). Metabotropic glutamate receptor subtype 2 is a cellular receptor for rabies virus. *PLoS Pathog*, *14*(7), e1007189. https://doi.org/10.1371/journal.ppat.1007189.

Warrell, D. A., Davidson, N. M., Pope, H. M., Bailie, W. E., Lawrie, J. H., Ormerod, L. D., Kertesz A, & Lewis, P. (1976). Pathophysiologic studies in human rabies. *Am J Med*, *60*(2), 180-190. https://doi.org/10.1016/0002-9343(76)90427-7.

Warrell, M., Warrell, D. A., & Tarantola, A. (2017). The Imperative of Palliation in the Management of Rabies Encephalomyelitis. *Trop Med Infect Dis*, *2*(4). https://doi.org/10.3390/tropicalmed2040052

Warrell, M. J., & Warrell, D. A. (2004). Rabies and other lyssavirus diseases. *Lancet*, *363*(9413), 959-969. https://doi.org/10.1016/S0140-6736(04)15792-9.

Whitehouse, E. R., Mandra, A., Bonwitt, J., Beasley, E. A., Taliano, J., & Rao, A. K. (2022). Human rabies despite post-exposure prophylaxis: a systematic review of fatal breakthrough infections after zoonotic exposures. *Lancet Infect Dis*. https://doi.org/10.1016/S1473-3099(22)00641-7.

Willoughby, R. E., Jr. (2015). Rabies: Rare Human Infection - Common Questions. *Infect Dis Clin North Am*, *29*(4), 637-650. https://doi.org/10.1016/j.idc.2015.07.006.

Willoughby, R. E., Jr., Tieves, K. S., Hoffman, G. M., Ghanayem, N. S., Amlie-Lefond, C. M., Schwabe, M. J., Chusid MJ, & Rupprecht, C. E. (2005). Survival after treatment of rabies with induction of coma. *N Engl J Med*, *352*(24), 2508-2514. https://doi.org/10.1056/NEJMoa050382.

Yamada, K., Noguchi, K., Komeno, T., Furuta, Y., & Nishizono, A. (2016). Efficacy of Favipiravir (T-705) in Rabies Postexposure Prophylaxis. *J Infect Dis*, *213*(8), 1253-1261. https://doi.org/10.1093/infdis/jiv586.

Zeiler, F. A., & Jackson, A. C. (2016). Critical Appraisal of the Milwaukee Protocol for Rabies: This Failed Approach Should Be Abandoned. *Can J Neurol Sci*, *43*(1), 44-51. https://doi.org/10.1017/cjn.2015.331.

Zhou, H., Zhu, W., Zeng, J., He, J., Liu, K., Li, Y., Zhou, S., Mu, D., Zhang, K., Yu, P., Li, Z., Zhang, M., Chen, X., Guo, C., & Yu, H. (2016). Probable Rabies Virus Transmission through Organ Transplantation, China, 2015. *Emerg Infect Dis*, *22*(8), 1348-1352. https://doi.org/10.3201/eid2208.151993.

Chapter 10

Poliomyelitis

Hayri Bozkurt*, MD

Department of Family Medicine, Heykel Family Health Center, Bursa, Turkiye

Abstract

Poliomyelitis, also known as "polio," is an acute infectious disease caused by an enterovirus that damages the anterior horn cells of the spinal cord and brainstem. Progress toward lower motor neuron cell death leads to the disruption of motor units and subsequent muscle weakness or complete paralysis. Although the virus is mostly eradicated in the western world, the postpolio decline is prevalent among people aged 60 and over. It is characterized primarily by fatigability and muscle weakness, but pain is also common. Reductions in lower limb muscle strength, voluntary drive, and endurance are likely to contribute to impaired balance control, a slow gait, and dysfunctional lower limb kinematics reported in polio survivors. Given these significant risk factors, polio survivors fall up to four times more often than their age-matched healthy peers. Interventions to improve function, reduce disability, and prevent falls in polio survivors are, therefore, clinically relevant, but studies are lacking, limiting the evidence base. Balance training, cognitive behavioral therapy, and the prescription of orthoses might be recommended. Muscle strengthening programs should be carefully designed and delivered due to their potential detrimental effects related to the excessive use and potential dysfunction of motor neurons and their axons.

Keywords: polio, vaccine, eradication, poliomyelitis, infectious disease

---

* Corresponding Author's Email: bozkurt_hayri19@hotmail.com.

In: Central Nervous System Infections
Editor: Mustafa Usanmaz
ISBN: 979-8-89113-660-1

Introduction

Polio (poliomyelitis) represents a disease caused by a poliovirus that attacks the nervous system. Children under five years of age are at the highest risk of having poliomyelitis. An enterovirus causes polio. The virus, taken into the body through the digestive system, is mostly transmitted in dirty environments and in the form of drinking dirty water, eating contaminated food, or hand-to-mouth contamination (Heymann, 2004). According to data from the World Health Organization (WHO), one in every 200 polio cases leads to permanent paralysis. Nevertheless, poliomyelitis has been eradicated in Europe, the Americas, Southeast Asia, and the western Pacific due to the global polio eradication initiative in 1988 (Halstead, 2011).

The polio virus, a highly contagious virus, is transmitted by contact with (infected) feces harboring the disease. Toys that contact or approach feces that contain the virus also carry a risk to children. Although very rarely, the virus can sometimes be transmitted by coughing or sneezing since the virus can survive in the throat other than the intestines.

People living in regions that have limited access to flush toilets or running water are at higher risk of being contagious because the feces of contaminated (infected or diseased) people can mix with drinking water in such regions.

People who have a more sensitive immune system, e.g., individuals with HIV infection, pregnant women, or young children, have a higher susceptibility to the poliovirus. In most cases, the only source is humans, and the disease occurs seven to 14 days after the virus is taken, but this period can vary between three and 35 days. People infected with this disease can spread the virus for ten weeks (2.5 months) and infect unprotected individuals during this period. The body eliminates the virus for weeks (ten weeks) with feces (Laffont et al., 2010).

Acute Illness

Of the cases, 60-70% occur in children younger than three years old and 90% in children under five years old. Most people infected with the poliovirus do not have any symptoms. About one in four infected people may have mild symptoms, including fever, nausea, weakness, nasal congestion, headache, sore throat, neck stiffness, cough, and pain in the legs and arms. The duration of the said symptoms is between two and five days in general. Afterward, they improve spontaneously. More significant symptoms affecting the brain and spinal cord are observed in a small portion of patients. As a result of the infection affecting the brain, permanent loss of muscle function in the legs and arms (the legs in general) or death may occur with loss of respiratory function due to the affected trunk and chest muscles. Paraesthesia (numbness and pins-and-needles sensation in the legs), meningitis (infection of the spinal cord and/or meninges in approximately one out of 25 individuals with poliovirus infection), and paralysis (inability to move the body parts or weakness in the legs, arms, or both in about one person out of 200 people with poliovirus infection) are observed. Paralysis represents the most severe polio-associated symptom since it can cause permanent disability and death (Marx et al., 2000; Nollet et al., 1999).

According to estimations, 95-99% of people infected with poliovirus are asymptomatic. The condition mentioned above is called subclinical polio. Although asymptomatic, poliovirus-infected individuals can spread the virus and pass it on to others without realizing it. Poliomyelitis can have non-paralytic symptoms, or if it reaches the nervous system, it can cause paralyzing (paralytic) symptoms (Querfurth and Swanson, 1990).

Symptoms of Non-Paralytic Polio

The duration of signs and symptoms of this type is between one and ten days. The following symptoms are observed with flu-like symptoms: Fever, sore throat, headache, vomiting, fatigue, and meningitis (Halstead, 2011).

Paralytic Polio Symptoms

About 1% of polio cases can develop into paralytic polio. Paralytic polio causes paralysis of the spinal cord (spinal polio), the brain stem (bulbar polio), or both (bulbospinal polio).

Paralytic polio has similar initial symptoms to those of non-paralytic polio. However, after a week, more serious symptoms will appear, including the following;

Loss of reflexes, muscle pain, and severe spasms, loose and drooping limbs (sometimes on only one body side), sudden paralysis (may be temporary or permanent), and deformed limbs (particularly the hips, ankles, and feet).

Complete paralysis is rare. Permanent paralysis is observed in less than 1% of all polio cases. The virus can cause death in 5 to 10% of polio cases (Laffont et al., 2010).

Diagnosis

It is possible to isolate the virus from the nasopharynx for five days. However, its isolation from the cerebrospinal fluid (CSF) or serum is rare. Elevated protein content and pleocytosis with normal glucose concentrations are observed in the cerebrospinal fluid. Nevertheless, the isolation of the virus is usually performed from the nasopharynx or stools. Molecular diagnosis with the polymerase chain reaction is currently the preferred technique to identify the poliovirus serotype and differentiate between wild and vaccine strain poliomyelitis (Kilpatrick et al., 1996; Muir et al., 1993).

Post-Polio Syndrome

A person who has had polio can still have a disease called post-polio syndrome (PPS) even after completely clearing the infection. It may occur within 15 to 40 years after the acute infection period. In general, post-polio syndrome is observed in 80% of people with polio infection (Trojan, 2005).

Common symptoms of post-polio syndrome (PPS) include (Kidd et al., 1997) the following:

- Progressive muscle and joint weakness, which may be unilateral or partial.
- Muscle pain gradually worsens: Pain increases with the increased amount of muscle use.
- Muscle wasting (muscle atrophy)
- Depression
- Difficulty breathing and swallowing
- Sleep apnea or other problems related to sleep
- Low tolerance to cold temperatures
- Fatigue is a common symptom that can occur as general fatigue or muscle fatigue.

- Concentration and memory problems (Gonzalez et al., 2010; Gandevia et al., 2010).

Halstead and Rossi described post-polio syndrome for the first time in 1987. It consists of three criteria: (1) the absence of other diseases that can explain a decrease in muscle strength; (2) new symptoms following a period of functional stability; and (3) a confirmed history of acute polio impacting the limbs (Halstead and Rossi, 1987).

Treatment of the Acute Attack

No drug can stop the polio virus or affect the virus directly. Hence, treatment focuses on improving the quality of life, coping with pain, and preventing possible complications. For this reason, vaccination is crucial before getting sick, and it is essential to ensure that children are vaccinated (Green, 1949).

The most common supportive treatments that can be performed while having polio are listed below as follows:

- Rest cure
- Pain relievers
- Antispasmodics for muscle relaxation
- Antibiotics for urinary tract infections
- Portable breathing devices (ventilators) assisting with breathing
- Physical therapy or splints to assist with walking
- Hot towels or hot water bags for the purpose of relieving muscle aches and spasms
- Physical therapy to control pain in impacted muscles
- Physical therapy for pulmonary and respiratory problems
- Pulmonary rehabilitation for increasing lung endurance
- If there is advanced leg weakness, a wheelchair or other mobility device may be required (Windebank et al., 1991).

Prevention

Cases of paralysis caused by polio are permanent and irreversible. It leaves lifelong sequelae and socially harms parents and individuals afflicted with the disease. It is very important to be protected from the disease because of the inability to work, restriction of movement, becoming an individual in need of support in society, not being able to perform every profession, being at risk of being isolated from society, being extremely disturbing, and death due to paralysis of respiratory muscles in very severe cases (Hall, 1992; Halstead and Rossi, 1985).

Vaccination is the best way to prevent poliomyelitis. There are two different vaccines for polio. The first is an oral polio vaccine (OPV = Live Vaccine) in the form of two oral drops, whereas the other is an inactive polio vaccine (IPV = Dead Vaccine) with intramuscular administration from the arm. The vaccine administered orally as two drops prevents the virus from causing the disease as a result of mixing with the blood from the intestines in the digestive system, whereas the vaccine administered from the arm provides a two-way and very strong protection by ensuring that protective substances against the virus are formed in the blood. The aforementioned double-sided protection application ensures that people stop infecting other individuals with the virus, leading to its complete ineffectiveness and disappearance (WHO, 2004).

The vaccination schedules of polio vaccines, which are also effectively applied in Turkey, can be summarized as follows:

- OPV: It is applied by administering two drops orally to infants who have completed their 6th and 18th months.
- IPV: It is administered in the 5-combined vaccine in the 2nd, 4th, 6th, and 18th months. This vaccine is administered intramuscularly. Intramuscular administration from the arm is performed once again in the 4-combined vaccine to children in the 1st grade of primary education, which is repeated a total of 5 times.

Side Effects of Poliomyelitis Vaccine:

- Oral Polio Vaccine (OPV): It should not be administered to those who have severe immune deficiency and are undergoing cancer treatment (especially leukemia cases). If there is a family member at home who is being treated for cancer, the same toilet should not be used. There is no harm in doing it when cancer patients and those receiving treatment do not need treatment and when their health conditions are suitable.

- Inactive Polio Vaccine (IPV): It has no known side effects, and there is no situation that should not be administered.

Healthy adults do not have a high risk of contracting the polio virus. There is the highest risk when traveling to a region where polio is still prevalent. Those who travel to such an area should be vaccinated.

The importance of vaccination emerges when we look at the number of cases observed over the years in the United States, which has implemented the vaccination policy actively and rapidly. Polio cases in the United States, which peaked at 57,623 cases in 1952, have continued to decline since the Polio Vaccination Assistance Act, and the disease was eradicated in 1979. In other words, no cases of polio have been observed in the US since 1979.

Conclusion

Although the incidence of new polio cases has recently been almost zero in developed countries and polio survivors are 60 years or older (people who contracted the virus in the 1940s and 1950s) (Gonzalez et al., 2010; Laffont et al., 2010), new polio cases remain unfortunately common in developing countries, meaning that the long-term impacts of this virus in those countries will continue for at least another 50 years, even at best. Although weakness, pain, and fatigue are sometimes seen alone after polio, the most important problem that causes a more troublesome picture is weakness and skeletal deformity. This weakness and deformity cause progressive orthopedic, respiratory, neurological, and general medical abnormalities in the future. It is important to know and explain that these symptoms, their disabilities, and their disorders are often treatable.

References

Fine, P. E. (2004). Poliomyelitis: very small risks and very large risks. *The Lancet. Neurology*, *3*(12), 703. https://doi.org/10.1016/S1474-4422(04)00928-7.

Gandevia, S. C., Allen, G. M., & Middleton, J. (2000). Post-polio syndrome: assessments, pathophysiology and progression. *Disability and rehabilitation*, *22*(1-2), 38–42. https://doi.org/10.1080/096382800297105.

Gonzalez, H., Olsson, T., & Borg, K. (2010). Management of postpolio syndrome. *The Lancet. Neurology*, *9*(6), 634–642. https://doi.org/10.1016/S1474-4422(10)70095-8.

Green, W. T. (1949). The management of poliomyelitis: the convalescent stage. In *Poliomyelitis: papers and discussions presented at the First International Poliomyelitis Conference* (pp. 165-185).

Hall, A. J. (1992). Polio eradication as 2000 approaches. *BMJ (Clinical research ed.)*, *305*(6845), 69–70. https://doi.org/10.1136/bmj.305.6845.69.

Halstead, L. S. (2011). A brief history of postpolio syndrome in the United States. *Archives of physical medicine and rehabilitation*, *92*(8), 1344–1349. https://doi.org/10.1016/j.apmr.2011.03.002.

Halstead, L. S., & Rossi, C. D. (1985). New problems in old polio patients: results of a survey of 539 polio survivors. *Orthopedics*, *8*(7), 845–850. https://doi.org/10.3928/0147-7447-19850701-06.

Halstead, L. S., & Rossi, C. D. (1987). Post-polio syndrome: clinical experience with 132 consecutive outpatients. *Birth defects original article series*, *23*(4), 13–26.

Heymann, D. L., & Aylward, R. B. (2004). Eradicating polio. *The New England journal of medicine*, *351*(13), 1275–1277. https://doi.org/10.1056/NEJMp048204.

Kidd, D., Howard, R. S., Williams, A. J., Heatley, F. W., Panayiotopoulos, C. P., & Spencer, G. T. (1997). Late functional deterioration following paralytic poliomyelitis. *QJM: monthly journal of the Association of Physicians*, *90*(3), 189–196. https://doi.org/10.1093/qjmed/90.3.189.

Kilpatrick, D. R., Nottay, B., Yang, C. F., Yang, S. J., Mulders, M. N., Holloway, B. P., Pallansch, M. A., & Kew, O. M. (1996). Group-specific identification of polioviruses by PCR using primers containing mixed-base or deoxyinosine residue at positions of codon degeneracy. *Journal of clinical microbiology*, *34*(12), 2990–2996. https://doi.org/10.1128/jcm.34.12.2990-2996.1996.

Laffont, I., Julia, M., Tiffreau, V., Yelnik, A., Herisson, C., & Pelissier, J. (2010). Aging and sequelae of poliomyelitis. *Annals of physical and rehabilitation medicine*, *53*(1), 24-33. *https://*doi.org/10.1016/j.rehab.2009.10.002.

Marx, A., Glass, J. D., & Sutter, R. W. (2000). Differential diagnosis of acute flaccid paralysis and its role in poliomyelitis surveillance. *Epidemiologic reviews*, *22*(2), 298–316. https://doi.org/10.1093/oxfordjournals.epirev.a018041.

Muir, P., Nicholson, F., Jhetam, M., Neogi, S., & Banatvala, J. E. (1993). Rapid diagnosis of enterovirus infection by magnetic bead extraction and polymerase chain reaction detection of enterovirus RNA in clinical specimens. *Journal of clinical microbiology*, *31*(1), 31–38. https://doi.org/10.1128/jcm.31.1.31-38.1993.

Nollet, F., Beelen, A., Prins, M. H., de Visser, M., Sargeant, A. J., Lankhorst, G. J., & de Jong, B. A. (1999). Disability and functional assessment in former polio patients with and without postpolio syndrome. *Archives of physical medicine and rehabilitation*, *80*(2), 136-143. https://doi.org/10.1016/S0003-9993(99)90110-7 .

Querfurth, H., & Swanson, P. D. (1990). Vaccine-associated paralytic poliomyelitis. Regional case series and review. *Archives of neurology*, *47*(5), 541–544. https://doi.org/10.1001/archneur.1990.00530050061013.

Trojan, D. A., & Cashman, N. R. (2005). Post-poliomyelitis syndrome. *Muscle & nerve*, *31*(1), 6–19. https://doi.org/10.1002/mus.20259.

WHO (World Health Organization) (2004). *Geneva declaration for the eradication of poliomyelitis*. Geneva: WHO.

Windebank, A. J., Litchy, W. J., Daube, J. R., Kurland, L. T., Codd, M. B., & Iverson, R. (1991). Late effects of paralytic poliomyelitis in Olmsted County, Minnesota. *Neurology*, *41*(4), 501–507. https://doi.org/10.1212/wnl.41.4.501.

Chapter 11

Tetanus

Yalçın Dicle*, **PhD**
Department of Medical Microbiology, Faculty of Medicine, Mardin Artuklu University, Mardin, Turkiye

Abstract

Tetanus is a fatal disease caused by tetanospasmin exotoxins produced by *C. tetani*, an anaerobic gram-positive bacterium. Although the disease can be prevented by vaccination, it is still a serious toxic fatal infection. While tetanus is less common in developed countries, it is a common infectious agent in less developed countries. The exotoxin tetanospasmin produced by *C. tetani* causes severe cramps, muscle spasms, and autonomic nervous system dysfunction in humans. Tetanus is usually caused by a contaminated wound, a skin rupture with compromised integrity, inadequate perinatal hygiene, or a cord cut with inappropriate materials during labor and delivery. To prevent tetanus, it is recommended that people of all ages be vaccinated with the tetanus toxoid vaccine to ensure good immunization. The rate of developing immunity against tetanus decreases significantly and inversely with age. The rates of developing immunity are quite high, especially in people who have been vaccinated for any reason in adulthood. Tetanus treatments generally aim to prevent muscle spasms and eliminate cardiovascular problems. In addition, if there is an open wound, the skin around the wound is cleaned, antibiotics and antitoxins are applied, and supportive care is applied.

Keywords: tetanus, infection, Clostridium tetani, vaccine

---

* Corresponding Author's Email: y.dicle65@gmail.com.

In: Central Nervous System Infections
Editor: Mustafa Usanmaz
ISBN: 979-8-89113-660-1

Introduction

Tetanus is a disease caused by a gram-positive, bacillary bacterium known as *Clostridium tetani. C. tetani* belongs to the Clostridiaceae family and is a motile, obligate anaerobe, life-threatening bacterium capable of forming spores. When stained with a g stain, they appear shaped like a tennis racket or a drum mallet. The bacterium is an anaerobic bacillus that produces a biological exotoxin called tetanospasmin, which can be fatal and causes tetanus, an acute disease characterized by spasms and stiffness in the musculoskeletal system (Weisberg, 2007). Bacterial spores are not completely destroyed in the sterilization process by boiling, but if sterilized in an autoclave at 120°C under 1 atmosphere pressure for 15 minutes, the spores can be destroyed. Tetanus is rarely cultured and is usually diagnosed clinically. Since *C. tetani* produces an effective exotoxin, this is generally how it produces its clinical effects. This bacterium can be isolated from human saliva, feces, feces of domestic animals, dust and manure, and can live anywhere its natural habitat is soil. It is a serious disease that causes illness if exposed to bacterial spores of *C. tetani* by any means (Mellanby & Green, 1981; WHO, 2018; Wilkins et al., 1988). Tetanus disease can often occur due to conditions such as surgical procedures, operations, penetrating injuries, tooth extraction, ear infections, bites, miscarriages, and post-pregnancy when the skin barrier is disrupted (Tezer, 2016). This bacterium can enter the human body and affect the central and the peripheral nervous system through wounds, deep cuts, and burns, or due to lack of hygiene in the perinatal period and lack of hygienic care of the cords of newborn babies. The majority of tetanus cases are caused by childbirth practices (Rhinesmith & Fu, 2018). Therefore, the toxins of the bacteria that enter the body in this way affect the muscles in the jaw and neck area, especially the painful spasms of the masseter muscles, causing muscle contractions that cause severe pain and an inability to open the jaw, also known as the "locked jaw" (WHO, 2018). In anaerobic environments, bacterial spores of *C. tetani* germinate into bacilli. Bacteria that transform into bacilli release exotoxins called tetanospasmin, causing muscle contractions and uncontrollable spasms. There are generally 4 forms of tetanus: localized, generalized, cephalic, and neonatal. While localized tetanus refers to muscle contractions seen mostly in the injured area, generalized tetanus can be defined as the classical form of this disease, it is seen systemically and is seen in more than 80% of patients. Cephalic tetanus is a form that results in cranial nerve palsy, which occurs mostly as a result of cranial lesions. In neonatal tetanus, it is a form that manifests itself with difficulty in feeding such as sucking and swallowing and is characterized by excessive crying bouts (Rhinesmith & Fu, 2018; Callison & Nguyen, 2021).

Epidemiology

Although tetanus can be seen in all age groups, this disease may cause more serious consequences in infants of mothers who cannot be protected with tetanus toxoid vaccine. Even though this disease is a particularly important public health problem, the incidence of the disease is quite high in underdeveloped countries or regions where vaccination policies and vaccine practices are inadequate and birth practices are carried out in unhygienic medical equipment and environments (WHO, 2018a). Tetanus continues to be more common in low- and middle-income countries, and although it is a rare disease in developed countries, it still constitutes an important public health problem (WHO, 2019). According to WHO reports, approximately 25,000 infants died in 2018 alone due to neonatal tetanus. These figures represent a decrease of approximately 88% compared to the rates of neonatal tetanus in 2000 (WHO, 2018a). The incidence of non-neonatal tetanus, on the other hand, has been gradually decreasing, and while the incidence of the disease was reported to be 0.21 per 100,000 in 1990, this rate was determined to be approximately 0.02 per 100,000 in 2006. According to the data from the Ministry of Health of the Republic of Türkiye, 161 of 923 cases of non-neonatal tetanus deaths and the mortality rate was reported as 17.4%, while 305 of 658 cases of neonatal deaths and the mortality rate was reported as 46.4%. According to the data of the Ministry of Health of the Republic of Türkiye, 199 cases of non-neonatal tetanus and 19 cases of neonatal tetanus were detected between 2007 and 2015 (Kurtoğlu et al., 2004).

It is difficult to understand exactly how widespread tetanus is. Most of the cases occur in underdeveloped countries with limited surveillance systems. Looking at the data of tetanus-related deaths worldwide in 2015, it is estimated that 79% of these deaths (44612) occurred in sub-Saharan Africa and South Asia (Kyu et al., 2017). It is thought that 18 people out of 100 thousand people worldwide, that is, approximately one million tetanus cases are seen in a year (Bleck, 2005). Since 1940, the incidence rate of tetanus disease has gradually decreased due to stable vaccination policies in developed countries and the use of antitoxin in wound treatment, and the incidence of the disease is approximately less than two per million. In particular, the development of countries has an impact on the incidence rates of tetanus. For example, in underdeveloped or developing countries, tetanus is a major cause of death in the neonatal group, whereas, in developed countries, it frequently occurs in adults who are not vaccinated or who are not adequately vaccinated. Sporadic cases are still seen in individuals who have not received any tetanus vaccine included in the new vaccine schedule (Pascual et al., 2003).

Vaccines and Immunization

The tetanus vaccine was first produced in 1924 during the Second World War to protect soldiers (Rhinesmith, 2018). Although tetanus is a disease that can be prevented by vaccination with tetanus toxoid, it is not possible to completely eradicate this agent because the tetanus agent is quite common. Therefore, in fact, efforts to reduce the incidence of the disease are aimed at elimination rather than eradication (WHO, 2019). Tetanus is a disease that can be transmitted to humans through minor or major contaminated injuries. Although this disease is caused by major injuries, more cases have recently emerged as a result of minor injuries. One of the most important reasons for this situation is that tetanus cases are more likely to be admitted to a health institution for major injuries and the given treatments are not interrupted, while for minor injuries, the current situation is not taken care of, and the treatment is neglected.

Since there is no routine adult vaccination program within the tetanus vaccination program in Türkiye, pregnant women, men to be recruited for military service, and adults in case of accidents or injuries can be vaccinated. For such reasons, it is stated that adults become susceptible to tetanus disease at an older age due to the decrease in antibody levels in people with primary vaccination problems caused by incomplete vaccination over time. In some cases, tetanus vaccination is given during childhood, but booster doses of the vaccine are often neglected, and the antitoxin levels of these people gradually decrease over time (Tosun et al., 2003).

Tetanus can be prevented with tetanus-toxoid-containing vaccines (TTCV), which are available in routine vaccination programs implemented worldwide and administered during pregnancy to protect the mother and baby. The WHO recommends at least 6 doses of the TTCV vaccine for lifelong protection against tetanus. At least three main doses and three booster doses are recommended. The first dose should be given at six weeks of age, and subsequent doses should be given at least four weeks apart. The booster doses are recommended between the ages of 12-23 months, between the ages of 4-7 years, and finally between the ages of 9-15 years. The ideal interval between booster doses is four years (WHO, 2018b). After all these vaccines, booster doses are recommended every ten years. The reason for this is the gradual decline in vaccine immunity. In a serologic study conducted in the United States between 1988 and 1994, it was reported that protective tetanus antibody levels were 72.6% after the age of 6 years, this rate increased to 91% between the ages of 6 and 11 years, titers dropped to around 47% between the ages of 20 and 70 years, and finally, tetanus antibody titers dropped dramatically to 31% at the age of 70 years and older (McQuillan et al., 2002).

Immunity does not occur naturally during tetanus disease, but antitoxin antibodies are formed in the sera of unvaccinated individuals, albeit at low titers. This is presumed to trigger subclinical toxin release from the gastrointestinal tract. It has been reported that serum levels of antibodies to tetanospasmin toxin are in the range of 0.01 U/mL and thus there are people with mild disease. As a result, immunity against tetanus disease can be achieved at around 100% with adequate dose vaccination.

Pathophysiology

Tetanus is usually caused by *C. tetani*, an anaerobic gram-positive bacterium sporulated in the soil. Although *C. tetani* is known to be present in human and animal feces, there are scientific doubts about its exact presence in human feces. In 1922, two researchers sought to answer this question by taking stool samples from 78 Chinese patients between the ages of 5 and 44 who were hospitalized with suspicions of various diseases and tested for the presence of *C. tetani* and found toxin-forming *C. tetani* in the feces of 26 (33%) patients (Tenbroeck & Bauer, 1922). In another study conducted in 1929, while no *C. tetani* agents were found in 100 adult human fecal samples, toxin, and non-toxin *C. tetani* agents were found abundantly in fecal samples taken from different animal species using the same method (Kerrin, 1929). The differences in findings between these two studies may be due to environmental conditions, occupational differences, inappropriate living conditions, and living in communal living areas with animals.

Conclusion

Tetanus is caused by an obligate anaerobic, gram-positive bacterium called *Clostridium tetani*. Tetanus is caused by a neurotoxin called tetanospasmin. Tetanus is less common in highly developed and educated societies but is more common in underdeveloped countries and societies with low levels of education. Tetanus is a disease that can be prevented and eliminated by vaccination. It is possible to prevent the disease with tetanus prophylaxis, proper infection treatment, and adequate supportive care. It is not possible for a person to be fully immunized even if they have tetanus. Therefore, children, pregnant women, and adults of all ages should be fully immunized. Immunization is possible at any age, and active immunization can reduce the incidence of the disease. In particular, the three main tetanus toxoid vaccines plus the recommended three booster doses can prevent the disease. However, since immunity titers decrease significantly over time, tetanus toxoid vaccination once every ten years after the last booster dose ensures that immunity remains at a higher level. Since tetanus is not transmitted from person to person, it is not possible to expect the development of herd immunity in the population. Although tetanus is not transmitted from person to person, studies have shown that tetanus develops under inappropriate conditions or as a result of some applications that penetrate under the skin such as earrings, piercings, and tattoos. Considering how common this situation is, it is understood how necessary and important lifelong immunization is.

References

Bleck, T. P. (2005). *Clostridium tetani* (tetanus). In: Mandell, G. L., Bennet, J. E., Dolin, R., (Eds). *Mandell, Douglas, and Bennett's Principle and Practice of Infectious Disease* (pp. 2817-22, 6th ed.). Philadelpdia: Elsevier, Churchill Livingstone.

Callison, C., & Nguyen, H. (2021). Tetanus Prophylaxis. In *StatPearls [Internet]*. StatPearls Publishing: Treasure Island, FL, USA. Available online: https://www.ncbi.nlm.nih.gov/books/NBK559008/ [Accessed on: 04.02.2023].

Kerrin, J. C. (1929). The distribution of *B. tetani* in the intestines of animals. *British Journal of Experimental Pathology*, 10(6), 370.

Kurtoglu, D., Gozalan, A., Coplu, N., Miyamura, K., Morita, M., Esen, B., & Akin, L. (2004). Community-based seroepidemiology of tetanus in three selected provinces in Turkey. *Japanese journal of infectious diseases*, 57(1), 10-16.

Kyu, H. H., Mumford, J. E., Stanaway, J. D., Barber, R. M., Hancock, J. R., Vos, T., Murray C. J. L. & Naghavi, M. (2017). Mortality from tetanus between 1990 and 2015:

findings from the global burden of disease study 2015. *BMC Public Health*, 17, 1-17. https://doi.org/10.1186/s12889-017-4111-4.

McQuillan, G. M., Kruszon-Moran, D., Deforest, A., Chu, S. Y., & Wharton, M. (2002). Serologic immunity to diphtheria and tetanus in the United States. *Annals of Internal Medicine*, 136(9), 660-666.

Mellanby, J., & Green, J. (1981). How does tetanus toxin act?. *Neuroscience*, 6(3), 281-300.

Pascual, F. B., McGinley, E. L., Zanardi, L. R., Cortese, M. M., Murphy, T. V. (2003). *Tetanus Surveillance-United States*, 1998-2000. Morbıdıty And Mortalıty Weekly Report CDC Surveıllance Summarıes. 52(3):1-8.

Rhinesmith, E., & Fu, L. (2018). Tetanus disease, treatment, management. *Pediatrics Review,* 39 (8), 430–432. https://doi.org/10.1542/pir.2017-0238.

Tenbroeck, C., & Bauer, J. H. (1922). The tetanus bacillus as an intestinal saprophyte in man. The Journal of Experimental Medicine, 36(3), 261.

Tezer, H. (2016). Difteri, tetanoz & boğmaca aşıları [Diphtheria, Tetanus & Pertussis Vaccines]. *Klinik Tıp Pediatri Dergisi*, 8(4), 27-32.

Tosun, S. Y., Atman, Ü., Kasırga, E., & İnceboz, Ü. (2003). Is the Booster Vaccıne for Tetanus in Older Age Necessary? *Türkiye Mikrobiyoloji Cemiyeti Dergisi*, 33(2), 148-52.

Weisberg, S. S. (2007). Tetanus. *Disease-A-Month*. 53(10):519-21.

WHO (2018a). *Tatanus*. https://www.who.int/health-topics/tetanus#tab=tab_1 [Accessed on: 04.02.2023].

WHO (2018b). *Prevention of Tetanus*. https://www.who.int/health-topics/tetanus#tab=tab_3 [Accessed on: 08.03.2023].

WHO (2019). *Maternal and neonatal tetanus elimination (MNTE)*. https://www.who.int/immunization/diseases/MNTE_initiative/en/index1.html [Accessed on: 08.03.2023].

Wilkins, C. A., Richter, M. B., Hobbs, W. B., Whitcomb, M., Bergh, N., & Carstens, J. (1988). Occurence of *Clostridium tetani* in soil and horses. *South African Medical Journal*, 73(12), 718-720. https://doi.org/10.1093/bja/87.3.477.

Chapter 12

Botulism

Yalçın Dicle*, PhD
Department of Medical Microbiology, Faculty of Medicine, Mardin Artuklu University, Mardin, Turkiye

Abstract

Botulism is a rare but serious illness caused by a toxin produced by the *Clostridium botulinum* bacterium. The toxin can cause paralysis and, in severe cases, it can be fatal. Botulism can be contracted through contaminated food, wound infections, or the use of contaminated drugs. Symptoms typically appear within six to 36 hours after exposure and include blurred vision, dry mouth, difficulty swallowing, and muscle weakness. Diagnosis is typically made through laboratory testing of blood or stool samples from a patient. Treatment involves administering antitoxin medication and supportive care to manage symptoms. Prevention measures include proper food handling and preparation, wound care, and avoiding the use of illicit drugs. While botulism is rare, it is a serious condition that requires prompt medical attention. Early diagnosis and treatment can improve outcomes and reduce the risk of complications.

Keywords: botulism, antitoxins, *Clostridium botulinum*, botulinum toxins

---

* Corresponding Author's Email: y.dicle65@gmail.com.

In: Central Nervous System Infections
Editor: Mustafa Usanmaz
ISBN: 979-8-89113-660-1

Introduction

Botulism is a rare but potentially fatal paralytic disease caused by the neurotoxin produced by *Clostridium botulinum*, a bacterium commonly found in soil and aquatic environments (Arnon et al., 2001). The toxin is one of the most potent neurotoxins known to man, and even small amounts can cause paralysis and respiratory failure. Botulism is a medical emergency and requires immediate treatment (WHO, 2018). The disease is characterized by muscle weakness, difficulty speaking and swallowing, and respiratory failure, which can ultimately lead to death (Feilchenfeldt-Maharoof, 2022). Rapid diagnosis and administration of botulinum antitoxin are among the main treatments for the disease (Shapiro et al., 1997).

The Centers for Disease Control and Prevention (CDC) has grouped biological agents that could potentially be used as bioterror or biological weapons agents into three categories (A, B, C) (CDC, 2019; Pınar, 2010; Serinken and Kutlu, 2009). According to this classification, agents (Variola Major (Smallpox), *Basillus anthracis* (Anthrax), *Yersinia pestis* (plague), *Francisella tularensis* (Tularemia), Filoviruses (Ebola, Marburg) (Viral hemorrhagic fever), Arenaviruses, *Clostridium botulinum* toxin (Botulism)) that carry a high degree of risk for national security are classified as Category A (CDC, 2019). These disease-causing or lethal agents, which can be turned into a powerful biological weapon with the help of low cost and simple technical support, have also started to be used as a threat by terrorist groups (Gökçe, 2001; Arnon et al., 2001). In this chapter, we will discuss the history, transmission and epidemiology, diagnosis and treatment, and prevention of botulism.

History

Botulism was first recognized as a distinct clinical entity in the late 19th century. Kerner was first clinically described in the state of Baden Württemberg in southwestern Germany. The disease was named sausage poisoning because it was thought to be caused by sausages made from pork. Later, in the mid-19th century, the disease was identified as 'botulus', a Latin word for sausage (Erbguth & Nauman, 2000; Torrens, 1998). In 1895, a German physician named Emile van Ermengem isolated the bacterium responsible for the disease and named it *Clostridium botulinum* (Van

Ermengem, 1979). The first outbreaks of botulism were linked to contaminated sausages in Europe in the early 20th century. Since then, botulism has been associated with a variety of foods, including canned goods, fermented fish, and honey (Peñuelas et al., 2022).

Transmission and Epidemiology

Botulism can be acquired through ingestion of contaminated food or inhalation of the bacteria's spores (Arnon et al., 2001). Foodborne botulism is typically caused by the consumption of improperly canned or preserved foods, such as vegetables or meat products that have been contaminated with *C. botulinum* spores (Centers for Disease Control and Prevention, 2022). Wound botulism can occur when bacteria enter an open wound and produce toxins (Sobel, 2009). Infant botulism is caused by the intestinal absorption of toxins produced by *C. botulinum* colonized in the intestines of children younger than 1 year of age (Arnon et al., 1981). In the United States, 80 to 100 cases occur each year (Shapiro et al., 1998). Since the normal intestinal flora of infants is not yet fully developed, it is thought that infants are more affected because they are not able to cope with the colonization of *C. botulinum* in the intestines. In this regard, some studies have reported that botulism originating from the intestines of infants is caused by honey consumed by infants under 1 year of age. Another proof that botulism is not only caused by honey consumed by infants under 1 year of age is that only 20% of infants with infant botulism consume honey (Spika et al., 1989).

Botulism is a rare disease in the United States, with an average of only 145 cases reported annually between 2010 and 2019 (Centers for Disease Control and Prevention, 2022). However, outbreaks can occur in certain populations, such as those who consume home-canned foods or use injectable drugs (Sobel, 2009).

Diagnosis and Treatment

The diagnosis of botulism is primarily based on clinical symptoms, with confirmation through laboratory tests of the patient's blood, stool, vomit, or food sample (Sobel, 2009; CDC, 1974). Early treatment with antitoxin, which binds to circulating botulinum toxin to prevent further damage, is crucial in improving the patient's chances of survival (Arnon et al., 2001). Supportive care, such as mechanical ventilation, may also be necessary to manage respiratory failure (Sobel, 2009).

Detection of the presence of *C. botulinum* in feces or wound material samples from an adult patient is generally considered sufficient to diagnose the presence of botulism. In infant botulism, the isolation of *C. botulinum* from materials is sufficient for a definitive diagnosis. However, there is a bioassay accepted as the gold standard test for the diagnosis of botulism. With this bioassay, it is aimed to determine whether the intraperitoneal toxin injected into mice reveals the symptoms of botulism. This standard biological test is performed in a small number of public health laboratories. In this test to determine the type-specific antitoxin, the detection of the antitoxin that provides protection usually gives results between 24 and 48 hours. However, this period could be even longer. Clinical management decisions are made accordingly (Sobel, 2005).

Botox

Botox, a pharmaceutical product derived from the bacterium *C. botulinum*, is injected into the human body for both clinical and cosmetic purposes. Treatments with this pharmaceutical product usually use diluted and purified botulinum neurotoxin type A. The neurotoxins type A, which are used in a very dilute form, are used in clinical settings in a manner and proportion appropriate to the patient's needs in Botox treatments. Although side effects can occur with Botox treatments, they can be tolerated in a short period of time (WHO, 2018).

Prevention

Prevention of botulism involves proper food handling and preparation techniques, including ensuring that canned foods are properly processed and stored, and avoiding the consumption of foods with bulging or damaged containers (Centers for Disease Control and Prevention, 2022). Individuals should also avoid using injectable drugs and seek medical attention for any open wounds that may become infected (Sobel, 2009). Prompt diagnosis and treatment, along with proper food handling and preparation techniques, are essential to prevent and manage this disease.

In the United States in the early 20th century, horse-derived botulinum antitoxin was administered in very high doses. However, despite this, the mortality rate of patients with botulism was still around 60-70%. Later, in the 1950s, a rapid decrease in mortality rates was observed, and finally, it is around 3%-5% today (Gangarosa et al., 1971). Antitoxin is not the only factor in this great decline, but the increase in quality of intensive care services brought by modern medicine has also been effective. Especially, the use of modern mechanical ventilation techniques and equipment can very effective. For this reason, patients with suspected botulism should receive supportive care services and, if necessary, should be hospitalized in an intensive care unit where mechanical ventilation can be provided. Patients with botulism may need to receive intensive supportive care services due to the very long duration of paralysis (Sobel, 2005).

Conclusion

In conclusion, botulism is a serious and potentially life-threatening illness caused by the bacteria *Clostridium botulinum*. It is contracted primarily through the consumption of contaminated food or by exposure to the toxin produced by the bacteria. Symptoms can range from mild to severe and, in some cases, can lead to paralysis and respiratory failure. Treatment for botulism typically involves the administration of antitoxin and supportive care, such as mechanical ventilation. Prevention is the key to avoiding botulism, and measures such as proper food handling and storage, as well as vaccination for those at high risk, can help reduce the risk of infection. Currently, there is no commercially available vaccine for *Clostridium botulinum*. However, there are ongoing research efforts to develop a vaccine for this bacterium. The primary way to prevent botulism is by practicing good food hygiene and avoiding consuming contaminated food or drinks. In addition, treatment for botulism usually involves supportive care and the administration of an antitoxin that can help to neutralize the botulinum toxin. Research is ongoing to develop a vaccine that can provide protection against botulism, but more work is needed before a vaccine is widely available. Prompt diagnosis and treatment are essential to prevent severe complications and death. While rare, botulism remains a significant public health concern, and prompt recognition and management are critical in achieving successful outcomes.

References

Arnon, S. S., Damus, K., & Chin, J. (1981). Infant botulism: epidemiology and relation to sudden infant death syndrome. *Epidemiologic Reviews*, 3, 45-66.

Arnon, S. S., Schechter, R., Inglesby, T. V., Henderson, D. A., Bartlett, J. G., Ascher, M. S., Eitzen E., Fine, A. D., Hauer, J., Layton, M., Lillibridge, S., Osterholm, M. T., O'Toole, T., Parker, G., Perl, T. M., Russell, P. K., Swerdlow, D. L., Tonat, K. & Eitzen, E. (2001). Botulinum toxin as a biological weapon: medical and public health management. *Jama*, 285(8), 1059-1070. https://doi.org/10.1001/jama.285.8.1059.

CDC (2019). *Botulism: Bioterrorism.* Available from: https://emergency.cdc.gov/bioterrorism/index.asp.[Accessed: 23.04.2023].

CDC (2022). *Botulism.* Available from: https://www.cdc.gov/botulism/index.html [Accessed on: 20.04.2023].

CDC (1974). *Botulism in the United States, 1899-1973: Handbook for Epidemiologists, Clinicians, and Laboratory Workers.* Available from: *https://stacks.cdc.gov/view/cdc/6673*. [Accessed on: 22.04.2023].

Erbguth, F. J., & Nauman, M. (2000). Letter to the Editor on the First Systematic Descriptions of Botulism and Botulinum Toxin by Justinus Kerner (1786-1862). *Journal of the History of the Neurosciences*, 9(2), 218-220. https://doi.org/10.1076/0964-704X(200008)9:2;1-Y;FT218.

Feilchenfeldt-Maharoof, S., Schaller, M. D., Berger, M. M., Tsouni, P., Kuntzer, T., & Ben-Hamouda, N. (2022). Foodborne botulism, a forgotten yet life-threatening disease: a case report. *European Review for Medical and Pharmacological Sciences*, 26(13), 4770-4773.

Gangarosa, E. J., Donadio, J. A., Armstrong, R. W., Meyer, K. F., Brachman, P. S., & Dowell, V. R. (1971). Botulism in the United States, 1899–1969. *American Journal of Epidemiology*, 93(2), 93-101.

Gökçe, G. (2001). Biyolojik Terör ve Biyolojik Savaş [Biological Terror and Biological Warfare]. *Sağlık'ta Nabız Dergisi*, 8(1), 16-39.

Peñuelas, M., Guerrero-Vadillo, M., Valdezate, S., Zamora, M. J., Leon-Gomez, I., Flores-Cuéllar, Á., & Varela, C. (2022). Botulism in Spain: Epidemiology and Outcomes of Antitoxin Treatment, 1997–2019. *Toxins*, 15(1), 2. https://doi.org/10.3390/toxins15010002.

Pınar, A. (2010). Biyolojik silah olarak mikroorganizmalar [Microorganisms as biological weapons.]. *Hacettepe Tıp Dergisi*, 41, 97-104.

Serinken, M., & Kutlu, SS. (2009). Biyoterörizm ve şarbon [Bioterrorism and anthrax]. *Türkiye Acil Tıp Dergisi*, 9(4), 185-190.

Shapiro, R. L., Hatheway, C., & Swerdlow, D. L. (1998). Botulism in the United States: a clinical and epidemiologic review. *Annals of internal medicine*, 129(3), 221-228.

Shapiro, R. L., Hatheway, C., Becher, J., & Swerdlow, D. L. (1997). Botulism surveillance and emergency response: a public health strategy for a global challenge. *Jama*, 278(5), 433-435.

Sobel, J. (2005). Botulism. *Clinical Infectious Diseases*, 41(8), 1167–1173. https://doi.org/10.1086/444507.

Sobel, J. (2009). Botulism. In Lutwick, S. M., & Lutwick, L. (eds), *Beyond anthrax: the weaponization of infectious diseases* (pp. 85-105). Humana Press.

Spika, J. S., Shaffer, N., Hargrett-Bean, N., Collin, S., MacDonald, K. L., & Blake, P. A. (1989). Risk factors for infant botulism in the United States. *American Journal of Diseases of Children*, 143(7), 828-832.

Torrens, J. K. (1998). *Clostridium botulinum* was named because of association with" sausage poisoning. *BMJ: British Medical Journal*, 316(7125), 151. https://doi.org/10.1136/bmj.316.7125.151c.

Van Ermengem, E. (1979). A new anaerobic bacillus and its relation to botulism. *Reviews of infectious diseases*, 701-719. https://doi.org/10.1093/clinids/1.4.701.

WHO (2018). *Botulism*. Available from: https://www.who.int/news-room/fact-sheets/detail/botulism [Accessed: 23.04.2023].

Chapter 13

Central Nervous System Parasites

Aydin Aydinli*, MD
Department of Medical Microbiology, Medical Faculty, Istanbul Okan University, Istanbul, Turkiye

Abstract

When parasitic infections of the Central Nervous System (CNS) are examined, we encounter quite a lot of parasites. Among protozoans, especially free-living amoebae (such as *Naegleria*, *Acanthamoeba*, *Balamuthia,* and *Sappinia*) have attracted attention in recent years. In addition to these, *Microsporidia* (*Encephalitozoon*), *Hartmanella*, *Malaria*, *Toxoplasma*, etc. will appear. It is important that different parasites are identified using different laboratory methods and their treatments are also different.

Keywords: parasite, central nervous system parasites, CNS parasite infections

Introduction

Free-living amoebae (*Naegleria, Acanthamoeba*, *Balamuthia*, and *Sappinia*) are particularly noteworthy within this group. In addition, well-known protozoa such as Malaria and Toxoplasma also cause parasitic infections of the CNS.

---

* Corresponding Author's Email: aydinaydinli@hotmail.com.

In: Central Nervous System Infections
Editor: Mustafa Usanmaz
ISBN: 979-8-89113-660-1

Free-Living Amoebae

Infections produced by small, free-living amoebae from the genera *Acanthamoeba*, *Naegleria*, *Sappinia, and Balamuthia* are not well understood or recognized clinically. In addition, most laboratories are unfamiliar with laboratory diagnostic methodologies for diagnosis. Some samples of these infections are primary amebic meningoencephalitis (PAM) -caused by *Naegleria fowleri*-, granulomatous amebic encephalitis (GAE) -caused by *Acanthamoeba* spp., and *Balamuthia mandrillaris*-; and amebic keratitis, cutaneous infections, and sinusitis -caused by *Acanthamoeba* spp-. Another newly discovered organism that has been linked to encephalitis was found. It has been established beyond a reasonable doubt that *Sappinia diploidea* is a human pathogen that was not previously known. The development of an efficient therapy for these diseases is still a problem. These free-living creatures get their sustenance from the bacteria and nutrients found in damp soil, freshwater, and seawater. The advent of diagnostic molecular approaches represents a distinct and possibly speedy method for identifying a few of these species not long after being cut off from their natural surroundings for the first time (Booton et al., 2003a; Booton et al., 2003b; Pasricha et al., 2003). Even though it is a well-established fact that free-living protozoa and pathogenic protozoa both host a diverse community of endosymbiotic bacteria, it is not understood what function these organisms play in the survival of the host, the infectiousness, or the invasion capabilities of the host. The investigation of free-living amebae's symbionts and parasites is in the preliminary phases at this point, and many of the words used to characterize these relationships are still evolving. In free-living amebae, there is serologic confirmation that some of the endosymbionts may be pathogenic to humans. This data has encouraged further research into the relationships between these two organisms. There is a wide variety of bacteria that are resistant to amebae; some of these bacteria are natural hosts of free-living amebae, others have been isolated from amebic amoebae, and yet others are resistant in vitro to a particular amoebic host. Some bacteria live their whole lives inside of cells, whereas others may choose to do so or not. Both types are classified as intracellular organisms. While some of these bacteria are well-known human diseases, others are new potential pathogens that were previously thought to be environmental species. Isolates of axenically grown *Acanthamoeba* have shown evidence of the presence of intracellular bacteria. *Naegleria* and *Acanthamoeba* amoebae may be infected with *Legionella pneumophilia,* which then causes the amoebae to multiply and eventually die. *Legionella* organisms, as well as other bacteria such as *Pseudomonas aeruginosa, Burkholderia cepacia, Burkholderia pickettii, Listeria monocytogenes, Campylobacter jejuni, Vibrio cholerae,* and *Mycobacterium leprae,* may be natural hosts for these amoebae (Axelsson-Olsson et al., 2005; Greub and Raoult, 2004; Marciano-Cabral and Cabral, 2003). It is believed that amoebic cysts serve as vectors for the transmission of these intracellular bacteria because of their well-known resistance to chlorine. This has huge implications for any healthcare facility where the water supply contains amoebae that are capable of free-living and surviving independently. There is additional evidence that the presence of amoebae in domestic water supplies may produce growth circumstances that enhance the pathogenicity of the organism to the human host. This is supported by the fact that residential water supplies contain amoebae (Thomas et al., 2004). *Chlamydia pneumonia*, echoviruses, and polioviruses can all be found in these amoebae (Greub and Raoult., 2004).

Naegleria Fowleri

In 1958, Culbertson et al. were the first to propose the idea that disease in humans could be caused by free-living amoebae present in water or soil, potentially leading to several diseases. Since then, there have been other occurrences of acute meningoencephalitis that have resulted in the patient's death (Schuster and Visvesvara, 2004a; Schuster and Vivesvara, 2004b). Nearly all the patients whose cases were recorded in the years shortly after this diagnosis of amoebic infections had a record of swimming in freshwater ponds or lakes for a short period prior to the onset of symptoms. This was the case for nearly all the patients whose cases were documented in the years immediately following this recognition of amoebic infections. This was the most common risk factor for contracting an amoebic infection. Only since the middle of the 1960s have infections of the CNS been recognized as being caused by free-living amoebae, and our understanding of the disease process that causes these infections is still insufficient. Meningoencephalitis, a subtype of the disease, is a severe condition that can result in death in a short amount of time. It primarily affects children and young adults. The condition shares many similarities with bacterial meningitis; however, it is caused by *N. fowleri*, an organism that thrives in environments with wet soil and fresh water. There have been close to 200 confirmed instances of PAM across the globe, with the United States reporting close to 90 of those confirmed cases.

It was believed up until recently that this virus was only seen in humans. However, infections have also been observed in a variety of different animals.

During its life cycle, the parasite goes through both the trophozoite and the cyst stages; however, the stage it enters is mostly determined by the conditions of its surroundings. Trophozoites can survive in artificial media such as tissue culture and can be found in moist soil or water.

Trophozoite Morphology and Structure of *Naegleria fowleri*: There are two distinct morphologies that can manifest as trophozoites: amoeboid and flagellate. It is possible to observe motility in hanging-drop samples made from cultures of cerebrospinal fluid (CSF), the amoeboid form, which is the only form that is known to exist in humans. This form is characterized by an elongated body with a broad front tail and a subsequent tapering tail. The diameter might range from seven to thirty-five micrometers. In most cases, the size of the round shapes is 15 micrometers. There is an exceptionally large karyosome present in the center of the nucleus, but there is no chromatin on the nuclear periphery. The granular appearance of the cytoplasm is due to the presence of vacuoles in it. When the amoeboid-form organisms are transferred from the culture into water or when they are tugged from the tissue into the water and the temperature is maintained between 27 and 37 degrees Celsius, they transform into a transient, pear-shaped flagellate form. The shift could happen relatively rapidly (within a few hours) or it could take up to 20 hours to take effect. The broad end of the flagellate shape is characterized by the presence of two flagella. Movement is typical and can take the form of both whirling or jerking movements. Some flagellate types are not divided; however, once they lose their flagella, they transform into amoeboid forms and resume reproduction.

Cyst Morphology and Structure of *Naegleria fowleri*. Cysts that are found in nature and those that are grown in agar cultures have the same appearance; each variety only has just one nucleus that is nearly the same as the nucleus as it is observed in the trophozoite. Typically, they are spherical, with diameters ranging from 7 to 15 micrometers, and have thick double walls.

Disease

A severe suppurative disease that affects both the meninges and the brain. It is known as amoebic meningoencephalitis, and it is caused by the bacterium *N. fowleri*. In humans, the disease results in death in a short amount of time, almost without exception. The amount of time that passes between the first encounter in conjunction with the organism, as well as the appearance of clinical signs such as rhinitis, headache, and fever, could range from two to fifteen days. Inhaling or aspirating water, dust, or aerosols that include trophozoites or cysts may also allow amoebae to enter the nasal cavity. This can happen when the amoebae are exposed to cysts or trophozoites. The parasite then travels to the cerebral cortex by way of the olfactory nerves after the invasion of the mucous membrane of the nose, most likely by phagocytosis of the cells that comprise the epithelium that surrounds the olfactory bulb (Schuster and Visvesvara, 2004). In addition to the above, creating an example of contact-dependent cytolysis that is carried out by heat-labile cytolysis with thermally stable hemolytic protein, and/or phospholipase enzymes (Schuster and Visvesvara, 2004a), the data show that *N. fowleri* consumes brain tissue directly through ingestion through the formation of suction saucers or amoebostomes. In most cases, cysts caused by *N. fowleri* cannot be seen in brain tissue. Early symptoms can include generalized discomfort in the upper respiratory tract, headaches, fatigue, and smell problems. In the acute phase, symptoms include a strong headache, a sore throat, and a stuffy, clogged, or discharge-producing nose. Nausea, vomiting, and stiffness in the neck are some of the progressive symptoms. Clouding of consciousness and coma are common symptoms in the last three to five days before passing away. In most cases, cardiorespiratory arrest and pulmonary edema are the factors that lead to mortality. It can be difficult to distinguish between PAM and acute purulent bacterial meningitis, especially in the earlier stages of either disease. PAM may be confused with acute purulent bacterial meningitis. Mainly polymorphonuclear (PML) leukocytosis, elevated protein concentrations, and reduced glucose levels are all characteristics that can be seen in the CSF of a patient with meningitis caused by bacteria. Unfortunately, when cerebrospinal fluid staining with gram is read wrongly, resulting in the identification of bacteria as a false positive, the antibiotic medication administered as a consequence has barely any effect on the amebae, and the patient frequently passes away within the first few days even though they take it (Schuster, 2002).

During the course of the amoebic invasion, extensive tissue destruction ensues. Ulceration can be seen in the mucosa of the nasopharyngeal, and the olfactory nerves are necrotic and inflamed at the same time. The area around the base of the brain and the olfactory bulbs shows signs of hemorrhagic necrosis in its most intense form. Meninges, perivascular spaces, and Sanguino purulent exudates are all potential harboring grounds for microorganisms. In 1997, the first recorded instance of organ transplantation from a donor who had passed away because of an undetected *N. fowleri* infection occurred. This research highlights the requirement for an appropriate examination of the advantages and hazards of giving tissues and organs for transplantation to people who may have received their ailments through contact with infectious substances. While none of the three organ recipients had future amoebic infections as a result of their transplants, this report highlights the necessity for such a review. It is understood that the Centers for Disease Control and Prevention are aware of another incident regarding a donor's kidneys being given away before it was established whether the person who donated the organ was found to have *N. fowleri* infection. There is no definitive answer about the potential transmission of N. fowleri via donor organs, and there is also no test that can be performed in a clinical setting to guarantee that donor organs are free from organisms. Furthermore, there is no recognized treatment protocol for transplant patients that uses preventive drugs.

Diagnosis

Because clinical and laboratory evidence can often not be used to distinguish, when trying to arrive at an appropriate diagnosis of pyogenic meningitis resulting from PAM, a procedure of exclusion may be required. To make an accurate early diagnosis, a high index of suspicion is often required. This is not always the case, despite most cases being related to exposure to polluted water through activities such as swimming or bathing. For the patient to have any chance of survival during the quickly deadly course that can last anywhere from three to 6 days following the onset of symptoms, quick identification and prompt treatment are required. The analysis of the CSF reveals lower quantities of glucose and increased concentrations of protein. The cell density of leucocytes may vary anywhere from a few hundred to more than 20,000 cells/mm^3. The Gram staining and culture results of cerebrospinal fluid (CSF) are both negative; nonetheless, the structure of the gram stain may be mistakenly interpreted as bacteria, which may result in the patient receiving inappropriate treatment.

The presence of amoebae in the CSF or in specimens obtained from a biopsy could provide conclusive evidence of the diagnosis. The cerebrospinal fluid or CSF that has been allowed to sediment should be placed on a slide, and then checked for the existence of mobile trophozoites. Smears can be additionally stained with Giemsa or Wright's staining. Light microscopy and phase-contrast microscopy are two types of microscopy that can be used to investigate CSF, exudate, or tissue pieces. It is essential to use extreme caution to avoid conflating leukocytes with living organisms or *vice versa*. Because of how easy it is to mistake leukocytes for amoebae, especially when one is investigating CSF using a counting chamber, it is recommended to use a simple slide and coverslip instead. It is possible for motility to differ, but the most distinguishing feature is the spherical nucleus that contains a large karyosome.

Before being examined, samples should never be chilled in the refrigerator. When centrifuging the CSF, it is important to utilize modest velocities (250 x g) to ensure that the trophozoites do not be spoiled. Even though bright-field microscopy with decreased light may be used, it is advised that phase microscopy be used instead if it is available. It may also be beneficial to use smears that have been stained with Wright's or Giemsa staining, or with a mixture of Wright's and Giemsa staining. In cases where *N. fowleri* is suspected of being the causal culprit, only the trophozoites are often observed. Patients with CNS infections may have cysts present in their samples if the infecting organism is *Acanthamoeba*. However, most cases are only identified after autopsies. The culture method and/or specific labeling with monoclonal antibodies using indirect fluorescent antibody (IFA) methods are required for validation of these tissue results. It is also possible to cultivate organisms on agar that do not contain any nutrients and are plated with *E. coli.*

Techniques such as indirect immunofluorescence and immunoperoxidase can be used in histological preparations in order to identify amoebae. The organism in tissue sections appears quite similar to a trophozoite of *Iodamoeba butschlii.* It contains a very large karyosome, but no chromatin, at the periphery of the nuclear envelope. It is also possible to identify the organisms by routine histopathological staining.

The periodic acid-Schiff stain gives a reddish hue to the cyst wall in cases when it is possible that *Acanthamoeba* spp. caused the infection, while the methanamine silver stain colors the cyst black. Both of these stains have the potential to be beneficial. Isolates of *Acanthamoeba* and *Naegleria* are often reference laboratories that may utilize indirect fluorescent-antibody approaches using a kind of monoclonal or polyclonal antibodies to identify organisms down to the species level. It is possible that the capacity of at least one of the epitopes to remain stable in formalin will be helpful in identifying *N. fowleri* in cemented samples obtained from biopsies and in studies pertaining to the state of the disease. In most cases, serological testing has not been of any use in making a diagnostic confirmation of this disease. The patient is unable to obtain an immunological response because the disease moves so quickly from stage to stage (Güeméz and Garcia, 2021).

Treatment

A large number of antibacterial and antiparasitic medicines have been tested for their ability to kill *N. fowleri* in both *in vivo* and *in vitro* settings. Although *N. fowleri* is quite susceptible to amphotericin B *in vitro*, only a small number of cases have shown signs of improvement after receiving intrathecal and intravenous injections of this medicine either alone or in combination with miconazole. There is recorded evidence of an instance in the United States in which a case was effectively cured with rifampin, miconazole, and amphotericin B. In vitro studies showed that the combination of miconazole with amphotericin B had a synergistic effect; however, rifampin was ineffective. This patient was also given dexamethasone and phenytoin to lower the patient's intracranial pressure and prevent more seizures, respectively. Infections caused by *Naegleria* have also been well cured with amphotericin B, oral rifampicin, and oral ketoconazole; amphotericin B alone; and amphotericin B, oral rifampicin, and chloramphenicol. It is unfortunate that there are so few survivors of PAM because *N. fowleri* is very sensitive to the antifungal medication with amphotericin B. There was a significant delay in diagnosis, which contributed to the fulminant character of the disease (Grace et al., 2015).

Epidemiology and Prevention

There have been close to 200 presumed or confirmed instances of PAM previously described among published works of science. These patients come from a variety of countries. Patients' clinical histories suggest that they were exposed to the organism just before the beginning of symptoms in swimming pools or freshwater ponds; prior to the beginning of symptoms, the instances were in good health and did not have signs of any specific diseases underneath. Individuals who had no history of contact with water have also had pathogenic *Naegleria* organisms isolated from their nasal passages, which points to the potential of an airborne exposure route.

The first environmental strains of pathogenic *N. fowleri* were reported in samples taken from soil and water in Australia, in addition to wastewater in

India, leading to the identification and isolation of the pathogen. There have been reports of the presence of *N. fowleri* in drainage wastewater that had been heated in both Belgium and Poland. Since then, more research publications have been published in which the authors discuss the process of isolating pathogenic or nonpathogenic isolates of *N. fowleri* from their natural habitats. Studies carried out in Belgium clearly show that *N. fowleri* strains exist in deliberately warmed waters (warm released from energy plantations), and investigations carried out in the United States showed that highly pathogenic isolates also exist in ponds in geographic locations with water conditions varying from 14 to 35 degrees Celsius that are entirely separated from any kind of heat discharging. According to these findings, the existence of virulent amoebic strains or isolates that have the potential to cause disease may depend not only on the weather but also on human intervention in the natural environment. Researchers from a number of different companies have been looking at the cysts' capacity for survival in a variety of different kinds of enviroment. According to these results, *N. fowleri* cysts that form during the milder summer months have a chance of surviving the colder winter months and have the potential to flourish during the summer months that immediately follow.

Education of the general population about the possible risks posed by polluted water is an important component of general preventive efforts. Because the DNA restriction fragment profiles of both environmental strains and human isolates are similar, it has been recommended that warm discharge water is not used for sports and recreational activities. This recommendation comes specifically from the discovery that environmental strains and human isolates have identical restriction fragment profiles. In more recent research, the randomly amplified polymorphic DNA (RAPD) approach was used to analyze thirty different strains of the bacterium *N. fowleri*. Previous research suggesting that RAPD variation is not associated with geographic origin was validated by the data presented here. In particular, the strains found in Mexico correspond to the variety that has been recognized in several other regions of the world, such as Europe, Asia, and the United States. The RAPD patterns that were produced by the strains in France were identical to those produced by the Japanese isolates. In addition to every single one of those strai, there is also a strain from France, which had characteristics that were comparable to those of strains found in the South Pacific. The findings demonstrated the existence of a large number of variations in European countries; however, just two different forms were discovered in the United States that were distinct from those found in South Pacific.

Acanthamoeba spp.

In the past, members of the genus *Acanthamoeba* were classified under the name *Hartmanella*. Sawyer and Griffin suggested a new family of spiny amoebae in 1975; they called it the *Acanthamoebidae*. The genus *Acanthamoeba* was designated as the prototype of the genus, and *Acanthamoeba castellanii* was designated as the prototype species. The presence of pseudopods that resemble spines and are known as acanthopodia is the trait that distinguishes this species from all others. The *Acanthamoeba* species; *A.culbertsonii*, *A.plyphaga*, *A.astronyxis*, *A.castellanii, A.divionensis,* and *A.healyi* are responsible for granulomatous amebic encephalitis, which typically affects immunocompromised, chronically unwell, or otherwise impaired individuals. These individuals often lack any relevant medical history that involves previous contact with recreational freshwater settings. *Acanthamoeba* spp. are also responsible for amoebic keratitis, and it is believed that there have been approximately 1,000 instances of *Acanthamoeba* keratitis diagnosed in the United States to this day. *Acanthamoeba* species such as *A.castellani*, *A.lugdunensis, A.rhysodes*, *A.quina*, *A.polyphaga*, *A.hatchetti*, *A.culbertsoni*, and *A.griffini* have been related to keratitis (Marciano-Cabral and Cabral, 2003). The incidence of *Acanthamoeba* keratitis appears to be fifteen times higher in the United Kingdom than in the US and sevn times greater than in the Netherlands (Kilvington et al., 2004), even though both countries have been seeing an upward trend in the total number of infections.

The principal classes of antibodies seen in serum are immunoglobulin M (IgM) and immunoglobulin G (IgG). Humoral immunity and activation of the complement system seem to be the key defensive mechanisms against *Acanthamoeba* infections. Phagocytic cells are more likely to recognize organisms when they are exposed to either antibodies or complement. Neutrophils, which are killed by amoebae, lymphokines act as a stimulant for cells, which causes them to accelerate the respiratory burst and liberate lysosomal enzymes. Lymphokines are responsible for this destruction. The most common forms of inflammatory cells that may be seen in tissues around amoebae are macrophages and neutrophils. In immunocompetent patients, the condition will progress to corneal opacity or perforation if treatment is not administered, despite the fact that neutrophils have invaded the cornea and a substantial humoral response has been observed. It was previously postulated that organisms conceal their specific antigens from the cellular immune responses, which would explain how they are able to limit the functions of macrophages and/or block the activity of neutrophils. Although there was no significant difference in the levels of total serum immunoglobulins between healthy individuals and patients with *Acanthamoeba* keratitis. The total blood immunoglobulins from healthy persons and patients with *Acanthamoeba* keratitis are quite similar to each other and do not substantially differ. Although *Acanthamoeba* infections are known to generate a granulomatous response, this reaction is either weak or nonexistent in patients with AIDS. The weak immunological response seen in these individuals is supported by these findings, which are in accordance with them.

GAE is a less well-defined form of meningoencephalitis that is generated by freshwater amoebae. It can manifest as a temporary or chronic disease, and it is characterized by the presence of localized granulomatous lesions in the brain. Hematogenous transmission is assumed to be the means by which pathogens reach the central nervous system; the major entry point is the skin or the lungs. In this particular disease, the lesions that occur in the CNS can include both trophozoites and cysts. It has also been found that a patient had a sudden beginning of symptoms including soreness in the neck, headache, and fever, which was followed by two days of feeling lethargic. There is a high probability that *Acanthamoeba* spp. are the pathogens responsible for most cases, but it is also likely that additional genera are involved. In the severe case that was discussed above, *A. culbertsoni* was detected in the CSF on many occasions and was cultivated from it. The patient showed a remarkable improvement after receiving treatment with a mixture of chloramphenicol and penicillin. Patients of GAE have been described in hosts with persistent disease or immunologically compromised; nevertheless, it seems that some individuals have neither a clear predisposing cause nor an immunodeficiency. Cancers, liver disease, infections caused by HIV (human immunodeficiency virus), SLE (systemic lupus erythematosus), skin ulcers, Hodgkin's disease, pneumonitis, renal failure, diabetes mellitus, pharyngitis, rhinitis, and tuberculosis are some of the diseases that are associated with smoking. These are some of the conditions that have been linked to GAE. Other conditions include rhinitis, pharyngitis, and TB. Alcoholism, drug misuse, treatment with steroids, hematologic diseases, systemic lupus erythematosus, pregnancy, acquired immune deficiency syndrome, chemotherapies and radiation therapies for malignancies, and transplants are all risk factors. Increasing numbers of acquired immune deficiency cases, especially individuals with low CD4+ counts, are being diagnosed with this disease as it becomes more common knowledge.

Keratitis and corneal ulceration are two more eye conditions that can be caused by the *Acanthamoeba* group. *Acanthamoeba* infection should be considered as a possible cause of ocular infections that do not respond to treatment with bacteria, fungi, or viruses, according to several reported cases that highlight the need for clinicians to take this factor into account when making a differential diagnosis. These infections are often caused by direct contact with contaminated materials or treatments intended for the eyes. It is now common knowledge that the use of contact lenses is one of the primary factors that contribute to the development of keratitis. Corneal scratches, incorrect contact lens maintenance, and the use of handmade saline solutions are all examples of situations that have been linked to disease.

Life Cycle and Morphology

Only the cyst and the trophozoite stages are present in the life period of *Acanthamoeba* spp., in contrast to *N. fowleri*, which has a flagellate stage.

Trophozoite Morphology and Structure

Motile creatures contain spine-like pseudopods; nonetheless, the progressive movement is typically not particularly obvious. The diameter of the trophozoites can range from 25 to 40 micrometers, with the average being 30 micrometers. The nucleus contains a typical example of a large karyosome, similar to the kind that occurred in *N. fowleri*. The structure in question is seen on a moist preparation. Such creatures rely on bacteria, algae, and yeast for sustenance in their natural environments; nevertheless, they are also able to subsist on liquid nutrients that they absorb by pinocytosis. Several of the organelles include rough and smooth endoplasmic reticulum, a Golgi complex, digestive vacuoles, mitochondria, independent ribosomes, and microtubules, which have been discovered and are commonly present in higher eukaryotic cells.

Morphology of Cysts

Cysts are typically spherical in shape and have only one nucleus. In addition to this, they have a large karyosome that is present in the nucleus of the trophozoite. It is common to be able to see the double wall, which consists of a slightly wrinkled exterior cyst wall and an interior cyst wall that has been characterized as polyhedral. The form of this cyst may be seen in organisms that have been cultivated on agar plates. The production of cysts takes place when environmental circumstances are unfavorable; cysts are able to withstand high temperatures between 0 and 2 degrees Celsius, chlorination, biocides, and antibiotics.

Diseases GAE

Acute suppurative inflammation of the brain and meninges may be the presenting symptom of meningoencephalitis brought on by *Acanthamoeba* spp., similar to what is seen in cases of *N. fowleri* infection. On the other hand, *Acanthamoeba* spp. is often known to induce a more chronic type of meningoencephalitis that is slow to progress and may last a long time. As a result of the misunderstanding that existed in the previous scientific literature on the names *Hartmanella* and *Acanthamoeba* spp., which were originally used for these species, they have been changed to be considered members of the same group as *Hartmanella* and *Acanthamoeba*. In human tissues, however, references to Hartmanella have to be changed to read *Acanthamoeba* or *Balamuthia* spp. (Kinnear, 2003). This is because it has been shown that no real species of *Hartmanella* is capable of causing disease in people.

It is not known how long the incubation period of GAE is; nevertheless, it is likely that the disease must be allowed to develop over a period of many weeks or months. Subacute or persistent manifestations are typical of the clinical course and are typically related to rather than to swimming, considered a traumatic event or chronic disease. Swimming is not considered a risk factor for this condition. Dizziness, confusion, sleepiness, vomiting, nausea, lethargy, headache, sometimes hemiparesis, seizures, and stiff neck are all symptoms of GAE. Within the CNS, both hemispheres of the brain are the components that are most likely to be impacted. There is the possibility of hemorrhagic necrosis and edema occurring within the temporal, parietal, and occipital lobes. It is possible to see a persistent inflammatory exudate covering the cortex, which is mostly composed of mononuclear cells and polymorphonuclear leukocytes. In contrast to PAM induced by *N. fowleri*, trophozoites, and cysts can be observed in many locations throughout the tissue. It has been discovered that the brain has granulomatous inflammation, necrosis, and thrombosed arteries. Granulomas composed of multinucleated giant cells may be found in individuals who are immune-competent, however, granuloma development is often poor or non-existent in immunocompromised people. It is not known whether direct destruction of tissue that is induced by organisms, the production of inflammatory cytokines such as TNF (tumor necrosis factor), interleukin-1, or both are the causes of brain necrosis. It is also possible for the infection to spread to other tissues in immunocompromised persons, including the liver, kidneys, trachea, and adrenal glands. Other less common sites of infection include both ears, as well as any necrotic bone that was harvested from the jawbone during bone transplantation.

Other space-occupying tumors that can be found in the CNS such as tumors, abscesses, fungal infections, etc., must also be examined in the differential diagnosis. Steroid treatment, alcoholism, diabetes, Hodgkin's disease, and pregnancy have been identified as potential risk factors for this condition. In addition to the adrenal gland, organisms have been discovered in the kidneys, liver, brain, pancreas, eyes, spleen, skin, uterus, and thyroid gland of humans.

An unexpected complication of having a bone marrow transplant is the possibility of developing amoebic meningoencephalitis. After undergoing autologous stem cell transplantation, a patient who was diagnosed with non-Hodgkin's lymphoma developed a case of the disease. Sixty-nine days after the transplant, the patient began to experience leg weakness, fever, and urine retention. Subsequently, the patient began to experience fever, convulsions, a rapid decline in mental function, and hypercapnic respiratory failure. The patient had a lesion that increased the size of rings at the level of the 11th and 12th thoracic spines, as seen by magnetic resonance imaging. It was observed that the CSF had pleocytosis. Following infection with *A. culbertsoni*, an autopsy revealed that the patient had subacute meningoencephalitis.

AIDS Patients

Even though the first instance of *Acanthamoeba* infection in an acquired immune deficiency syndrome case was not published until 1986, there have been a significant number of further cases documented since then. It is already good knowledge that some species of *Acanthamoeba* can cause opportunistic infections in immunocompromised people living with acquired immune deficiency syndrome. However, the vast majority of the incidents have ended in fatalities, which have been verified post-mortem. These people often have a more advanced stage of HIV infection and a very low CD4+ T-cell count, typically less than 200/mm^3. Most of the time, patients pass away within a month after the start of CNS symptoms. Unfortunately, to correctly diagnose this illness, a high index of suspicion is required. This is due to the possibility that physiological and histological signs might be similar to those associated with a common fungal or algal disease. It is believed that the infection spreads first to the lungs and then to the sinuses. There is speculation that the skin itself might serve as an access point. Chills and fever, neurologic symptoms or nasal congestion, musculoskeletal, and skin lesions are some examples of the types of general problems that might be present. People who have AIDS are more likely to develop erythematous nodules, persistent ulcerative lesions, and abscesses of the skin, than other people. Despite CSF lymphocytosis being seen in people who do not have AIDS, the CSF of HIV-positive patients may not display any cells at all. In addition to that, they often have chronic sinusitis, otitis, and skin diseases. Notwithstanding the fact that serologic testing for toxoplasma can come out negative in people who have neurological symptoms and AIDS, the condition of toxoplasmosis may be incorrectly diagnosed in these patients. Other individuals have received an incorrect diagnosis of bacterial meningitis, squamous cell cancer, or vasculitis of the central nervous system.

Patients who arrive with acceptable histories and imaging results, such as nonspecific cerebral edema on CT in the event of PAM and localized punctate-enhancing lesions in the posterior cranial fossa on T1-weighed MRI in the case of GAE, are considered to be in a better position to diagnose the condition. They should have both PAM and GAE considered in the differential diagnosis of their condition, despite the fact that both conditions are thought to be rare. Both conditions also have a grave prognosis. In most cases, the first symptoms that appear are a temperature and headache. It is essential to keep in mind that a review of cranial computed tomography in patients with toxoplasmosis is unable to differentiate between the two potential causal factors, *Acanthamoeba* and/or *Toxoplasma*. This is something to keep in mind. In patients who have spread the disease, the amount of time between the beginning of the infection and the patient's passing might vary anywhere from seven days to five months. After the neurologic signs have become apparent, the average amount of time a person may survive is approximately a month. The importance of recognizing this condition as a possible cause of the patient's presentation cannot be overstated. Earlier treatment has been shown to improve clinical outcomes. It is critical to conduct the right diagnostic tests as quickly as possible in order to determine the agent that is the source of the problem.

Keratitis

There has been a correlation established between *Acanthamoeba* spp. and corneal ulcers, keratitis, and uveitis. Infections have been obvserved in people using soft and hard lenses, and a particular emphasis has been placed on the disinfection techniques for soft lenses, including homemade saline treatments. When it comes to the elimination of *Acanthamoeba* trophozoites and cysts, it seems that heat disinfection is, on average, more efficient than cold disinfection approaches. Recent research has shown that not all commercial contact lens disinfection solutions have the same level of effectiveness in killing microorganisms *A.castellanii* (Beattie et al., 2003). Both trophozoites and cysts were susceptible to the killing effects of solutions that included either hydrogen peroxide or chlorhexidine-thimerosal. Only trophozoites were susceptible to the killing effects of a solution based on benzalkonium chloride, but solutions that included poly aminopropyl biguanide or polyquaternium-1 were absolutely ineffective.

Cutaneous Lesions

Regardless of whether there is involvement in the central nervous system or not, persons with AIDS are more likely to have cutaneous lesions. The condition is characterized by the appearance of firm skin ulcers or erythematous nodules. The first lesions manifest as hard popular nodules that discharge purulent fluid; these lesions develop into indurated ulcers later on. that do not heal. It is not known whether skin lesions reflect a central focus or whether they may be the consequence of hematogenous spread from other body locations, despite the fact that there is a possibility that widespread skin lesions are the initial sign of an illness caused by *Acanthamoeba*. Despite the fact that the mortality rate for these individuals without central nervous system involvement is approximately 75%, the mortality rate increases to 100% when skin infection is accompanied by central nervous system diseases. This is because the risk of infection in the CNS is much higher than the risk of infection in the skin. Histology indicates vasculitis, trophozoites, and necrosis surrounded by inflammatory cells. Amoebae cysts and trophozoites are also seen. On the other hand, similar results may potentially be confused with skin lesions caused by fungi, viruses, mycobacteria, or responses to foreign bodies. The yeast forms of *Blastomyces dermatitidis*, *Cryptococcus neoformans*, sporangia of *Rhinosporidium seeberi*, or *Prototecha wickerhamii* may also resemble amoebae. The skin condition known as cutaneous acanthamoebiasis has been misidentified as a variety of different conditions on several occasions; if the first results are inconclusive and no amoebae are discovered, it is required to reevaluate the biopsy material using a new specimen and the procedure again. This is due to the fact that cutaneous acanthamoebiasis has been incorrectly identified as a variety of other diseases.

Diagnosis

These organisms can be recovered and identified using laboratory tests that are comparable to those used for *N. fowleri*. The only exception to this is the recovery method of culture, which has not been shown to be as successful in cases of granulomatous amebic encephalitis infected with *B.mandrillaris*. The use of non-nutrient agar plates with Page's saline and a growth of *Escherichia coli* that is superimposed, from which the anemones consume food from, is the method that has been shown to be the most successful. Phosphate-buffered saline is another option that has been shown to be viable. In addition, samples that have been carried in amoeba-saline (5.0 ml) and filtered using cellulose acetate and nitrate filters measuring 13 millimeters in diameter and 0.22 micrometers in pore size have been considered suitable for organism recovery. After that, the filter is positioned in the exact middle of the non-nutrient agar plate that has *E. coli* planted on it. Cysts might be stained with calcofluor white, periodic acid-Schiff, and Gomori's silver methenamine, which are all good tissue stains.

There have been other formulations of the enhanced medium that have been produced, providing some more choices. *Acanthamoeba* isolates have been isolated from samples after being inoculated on tryptic soy agar containing 5% sheep or horse blood, non-nutrient agar with *E. coli* (live or dead bacteria) and buffered charcoal-yeast extract (BCYE) agar, respectively. Healthy healing of cysts was achieved using TSA with either horse blood or rabbit blood. However, only non-nutrient agar containing live *P. aeruginosa* and live *E. coli* produced a good recovery of trophozoites. This was true for all bacterial species, whether dead or alive (*Klebsiella pneumonia*, *E. coli*, *Enterobacter aerogenes*, *Serratia marcescens*, *Pseudomonas aeruginosa*,

Stenotrophomonas maltophilia, and *Staphylococcus aureus*). The optimal recovery of *Acanthamoeba* was achieved using TSA with horse blood or rabbit blood, non-nutrient agar, and BCY agar inoculated with live *S. maltophilia, P. aeruginosa,* or *E. aerogenes.*

Studies on cryopreservation have also shown that the trophozoites of *A. culbertsoni* have the maximum viability when the final concentration of dimethyl sulfoxide is maintained at 10% and the ideal warmth is maintained at 4°C. When trophozoites were thawed from a frozen suspension, no obvious cultural or morphological changes were seen in the organisms (Alejandre-Aguilar et al., 1998). The organisms were cultivated on a medium consisting of serum, casein, glucose, and yeast extract.

Even for expert microscopists, it may be difficult to identify *Acanthamoeba* in the eye and other tissues. It seems that organisms, when histologically prepared, are extremely comparable to keratoplasty, including monocytes and leukocytes. According to an estimate, up to seventy percent of clinical cases of *Acanthamoeba* keratitis are considered to be misinterpreted as having viral keratitis. Patients who have GAE or respiratory symptoms may have cytospin preparations made from their CSF or bronchoalveolar lavage fluid (BAL). When hematoxylin-eosin or trichrome stains are used in fixed preparations that have been produced by cytocentrifugation, the distinctive features of *Acanthamoeba* trophozoites, such as the prominent nucleolus, contractile vacuole, and cytoplasmic vacuoles, can be observed with greater clarity. This is because the trophozoites have been fixed.

Even though it has been shown that antibodies to *Acanthamoeba* spp. may be detected, it has not been demonstrated that serologic testing is helpful in the identification of these diseases (Schuster, 2002).

Treatment Disseminated Infections

There is a wide range of susceptibility among *Acanthamoeba* isolates' trophozoites and cysts to various antimicrobial drugs. *In vitro* tests have shown that they are susceptible to treatment with pentamidine, ketoconazole, paromomycin, hydroxystilbamidine, polymyxin, 5-fluorocytosine, trimethoprim-sulfamethoxazole, azithromycin, and sulfadiazine preparations of medicinal herbs; in particular, they are susceptible to combinations of these medications. Greater awareness of these diseases and the initiation of treatment at an early stage are two factors that significantly impact the results for patients. In earlier times, steroids were used to treat cerebral inflammation and edema in patients who suffered with CNS diseases; however, this treatment strategy should not be employed as steroids have a tendency to make the *Acanthamoeba* infection worse. In earlier times, steroids were used to treat brain inflammation and edema in patients with CNS diseases. Antimicrobial combinations, such as those consisting of pentamidine isethionate, sterol-targeting azoles (miconazole, clotrimazole, fluconazole, itraconazole, ketoconazole), sulfadiazine, and 5-fluorocytosine, have been used to treat encephalitis. These treatments have had some degree of effectiveness. Combining medications is an effective way to combat drug resistance, which may already exist or develop throughout therapy. *In vitro*, research has shown that different strains and species are sensitive to different drugs, yet a single drug has been shown to be effective against all amoebae (McBride et al., 2005).

Epidemiology and Prevention

The basic preventive actions are pretty similar to those adopted for *N. fowleri* before. It has been shown that a number of disinfectants are effective contrary to both *Acanthamoeba and Naegleria* spp. In general, the finding is that *Naegleria* spp. are vulnerable to the amounts of chlorine seen in swimming pools, but *Acanthamoeba* species are more vulnerable to the chemical than other types of bacteria. The discovery of *Acanthamoeba* spp. in pharyngeal and nasal isolates may be evidence that the organisms were brought to swimming pools by humans. There are undoubtedly a variety of variables that contribute to the increasing frequency of infection, including a significant amount of people have been affected by the human immunodeficiency virus (HIV), as well as an increased number of patients receiving chemotherapy for cancer or immunosuppressive medication for organ transplantation. At a temperature of 4 degrees Celsius, *Acanthamoeba* cysts can maintain their ability to reproduce for up to 24 years. It was not until after eight years of in vitro culture that some of the isolates had entirely lost their virulence, as proven by research conducted on animals.Based on these findings, it is reasonable to conclude that the viability of cysts can reach 25 years and that they may keep their invasive capabilities during this time. The main risk factors for *Acanthamoeba* keratitis include not disinfecting daily-wear soft contact lenses and employing chlorine-release lens disinfection systems, both of which have limited effecacy against the organism. *Acanthamoeba* is the pathogen that causes keratitis, which is an infection of the cornea (Garcia, S. L., 2007).

Balamuthia Mandrillaris

It was previously believed that the free-living amoeba *Balamuthia mandrillaris* was just another innocuous soil organism and that it did not or could not infect mammals. However, recent research has shown that this is not the case. Nevertheless, because *B. mandrillaris* was initially identified in a pregnant mandrill at the San Diego Wild Animal Park that had died of meningoencephalitis, a variety of primate species, including gibbons, gorillas, orangutans, monkeys, and baboons, as well as a horse and, a sheep, have died of CNS infection caused by this organism. Other animals that have succumbed to this infection include sheep and a horse. Up to 90 cases of human amoebic encephalitis have been reported around the world, and approximately 19 of those cases have been diagnosed in the United States. After the development of symptoms similar to those of a stroke, which may be confused with those of other diseases such as the brain stem glioma, death can occur anywhere between one week and many months later. Patients ultimately die as a result of severe CNS disease. One person who survived the virus was left with profound brain damage.

Life Cycle and Morphology

In contrast to organisms classified as *N. fowleri*, *Balamuthia mandrillaris* does not go through a period in the course of its life in which it produces flagella; instead, the life cycle of *Balamuthia mandrillaris* is comparable to that of *Acanthamoeba* spp.

Trophozoite Morphology and Structure of *B. mandrillaris*

Trophozoites produced by *B. mandrillaris* are often characterized by an uneven form, and the length of actively feeding amoebae may range from twelve to sixty μ (the average being 30 μ). When the monolayer cells of tissue culture are disrupted, the trophozoites produce pseudopodia in the shape of fingers, in contrast to the broad pseudopodia that are often seen in tissue culture.

Cyst Morphology and Structure of *B. mandrillaris*

Cysts are typically spherical in shape and range in diameter from 6 to 30 micrometers. When examined with an electron microscope, the cysts are distinguished by the presence of three layers inside the wall of each cyst. These layers are as follows: an outside stretchy ectocyst, a structureless mesocyst in the center, and a thin endocyst on the inside of the cyst. It seems like they have two walls when seen with a light microscope; the outside wall is more irregular, while the inner wall is more spherical.

Disease

The incubation time of this disease, which is quite similar to GAE and is caused by *Acanthamoeba* species, is unclear. The signs and symptoms of the disease are often intermediate or persistent, and swimming in freshwater is generally not associated with it. There are no single diagnostically useful clinical symptoms, laboratory results, or radiologic signs that have been identified for GAE. The results of the neuroimaging study show that the lesions are diverse, hyperdense, non-enhancing, and space-occupying (Schuster, 2002).

They mostly affect the cerebral cortex and the subcortical white matter, regardless of whether they are single or numerous. These results point to the possibility of a tumor in the central nervous system, septic infarcts, or tuberculoma.

Nausea, headaches, fever, vomiting, dysphagias, visual abnormalities, hemiparesis, and seizures are some of the symptoms that patients report experiencing. The clinical course may also vary greatly from patient to patient, lasting anywhere from a few days to many months at a time.

Amoebae are surrounded by macrophages, lymphocytes, and neutrophils when they are in immunocompetent hosts. This indicates that an inflammatory response has been initiated, with very rare exceptions, these individuals also often pass away as a result of serious CNS disease. In many of the same tissues of the CNS that contain trophozoites and cysts of *Acanthamoeba* spp., *B.*

mandrillaris can also be identified. Although it is difficult to differentiate these two species in tissue using light microscopy, *B. mandrillaris* seems to contain more than one nucleus in the nucleus in certain tissue portions. In most cases, the final identification of *B.mandrillaris* requires the use of electron microscopy in conjunction with histochemical techniques. The most accurate method of differentiating between *Acanthomoeba* and *Balamuthia* spp. is an immunoflorence test that uses sera that are unique to the respective species (Kum et al., 2019).

Diagnosis

It is important to highlight that the attempts made to eliminate the organisms from some people affected by GAE have not been effective. Furthermore, in non-nutrient agar plates that were planted with *E. coli*, it has been shown that *B. mandrillaris* does not grow as well as it does on other types of agar. These organisms can be cultivated in mammalian cell cultures in the diagnostic laboratory; it has been shown that monkey cells of the kidney, as well as MR, diploid macrophage cell lines, and HEp-2 have been shown to be used to achieve a certain level of success. Researchers were able to cultivate it, using human brain microvascular endothelial cells, culture *B. mandrillaris* obtained postmortem from the brain, and CSF of a patient with granulomatous amebic meningoencephalitis (Jayasekera et al., 2004). There is also now a cell-free growing medium that may be purchased. The trophozoites are distinguished by their considerable branching and solitary nucleus (although it is possible to see binucleate forms on occasion) that is surrounded by karyosomes. On occasion, one or two elongated forms include a significant number of contractile vacuoles, as will be shown. The cysts contain only one nucleus inside them (although it is possible to find binucleate variants within them on occasion), and they have the typical double wall structure, with the outer wall seeming thick and uneven.

Adults and children have been reported to have antibodies in their serum that are directed against *B. mandrillaris*; however, testing that can be used routinely is not yet accessible. Mice that have been infected with *Acanthamoeba* spp. or *B.mandrillaris* may die of the acute disease within five to seven days, or from chronic disease after many weeks. This is despite the mouse model being used seldomly, since it is considered to be quite impractical. In either situation, culture or a histologic study of the mouse brain will reveal the presence of amoebae in the organ.

Primers that generate a PCR product that is particular to *Balamuthia mandrillaris* have been created as a result of the sequence analysis of the genes that make up the mitochondrial small-subunit rRNA. Not only will these primers be valuable considering the past examinations of tissues that have been kept, but they will also be beneficial for the potential verification of organisms *in vivo* (Booton et al., 2003b). According to research on genotyping, the potentially fatal infections caused by *B. mandrillaris* are caused by a single species that can be found throughout the world. It would seem that there is no correlation between the genus of an animal and a particular mitochondrial sequencing that is infected with the virus.

Treatment

It has been shown through in vitro research that pentamidine isethiocyanate is effective against *B. mandrillaris*; therefore, it is reasonable to hypothesize that patients who are afflicted with this condition may benefit from the use of this drug. The antiamoebic capabilities of ketoconazole, propamidine isethionate, lotrimazole, and some biguanides have been found to be shown by the results of previous research (Jung et al., 2004; Schuster and Visvesvara, 2004; Siddiqui et al., 2022). The one immunocompetent patient who was able to survive therapy was treated with a combination of antibiotics (sulfadiazine, pentamidine, clarithromycin, and fluconazole) (Kinnear, 2003). This patient was able to survive treatment. In order for the patient to continue to live, medicine was administered.

Epidemiology and Prevention

The most recent recommendations are very comparable to those for *Acanthamoeba* species and species-related variants. There is very little information available on the state of the environment in which *B. mandrillaris* lives; nevertheless, it is generally accepted that the natural environment is comparable to that of other amoebae that are free-living. Despite the fact that efforts to isolate *B. mandrillaris* from soil associated with previous occurrences of encephalitis were unsuccessful. Nevertheless, after the death of a child in northern California who was 3 years old from amoebic encephalitis caused by *Balamuthia mandrillaris*, soil samples were collected near the child's house and in the regions outside where the child played. An amoeba exhibiting characteristics typical of *Balamuthia* was extracted from the soil discovered in the restricted space of a plant inside the house (Schuster et al., 2003). As a result, the confirmation of *Balamuthia*'s identity as a free-living amoeba may be achieved by its isolation from the soil. Similar to *Balamuthia, Naegleria*, and *Acanthamoeba,* and it is an opportunistic pathogen.

In light of the material provided so far, it is abundantly obvious that *B. mandrillaris*, which was once thought to have limited infectious potential, continues to be accepted as the primary cause of lethal meningoencephalitis in both humans and animals. This recognition is likely to persist for some time. It is possible that people living with AIDS may continue to be ill as a result of this opportunistic disease.

Sappinia Diploidea

Amebic encephalitis is a condition that may be caused by a recently discovered human infection called *Sappinia diploidea*. One patient has provided sufficient evidence that the infection is present (Gelman et al., 2003). The sizes of trophozoites can vary from 40 to 70 μ and include a double nucleus that is easily identifiable. The trophozoites have two nuclei, and transmission electron microscopy has shown that these nuclei are linked to each other by connecting filaments that are perpendicular to each other. The Giemsa and periodic acid-Schiff stains revealed that the trophozoites consumed host blood cells and had produced a brilliant stain. Although cysts were not seen, it cannot be ruled out that they are present in the human host. *S. diploidea* was identified as a human pathogen for the first time because of these and other morphologic characteristics that were necessary for the diagnosis.

The patient was a male in his 38th year who presented with complaints of visual abnormalities and headaches, as well as an episode of seizure activity. The posterior left temporal lobe of the patient's brain had a single mass with characteristics of malignancy. The tissue sample taken from the mass revealed necrotizing hemorrhagic inflammation, and it also included amebae that were still alive. Following surgery, the patient received a series of antiamebic medications of the order of azithromycin, pentamidine, itraconazole, and flucytosine as part of their postoperative care (Visvesvara et al., 2007).

Microsporidia

Although *Microsporidia* are classified as real eukaryotes, they also exhibit molecular and cytological traits that are more typical of prokaryotes. These characteristics include elements of the translational machinery and genome size that fall within the range of bacteria. Furthermore, *Microsporidia* do not have any mitochondria, peroxisomes, or Golgi membranes that are easily recognized (Mansfield and Gajadhar, 2004). Phylogenetic analyses have shown beyond a reasonable doubt that the microsporidia were generated by the fungus and had the strongest ties to the zygomycetes. A number of other characteristics, such as the existence of trehalose and chitin, similarity in cell cycle processes, and also specific genome organizational patterns, are shared with fungi. *Microsporidia* are currently regarded to be highly specialized fungi that have endured functional and genetic distortions, leading to the creation of one of the smallest eukaryotic genomes that exist. This is due to the fact that microsporidia have lost their ability to produce spores. Nevertheless, at this juncture in history, diagnostic and clinical concerns and obligations might still be left with these organisms and the parasitologists will continue playing a role in the work that is being done in the field of parasitology. It is possible that we are at a transitional period, comparable to what happened with *Pneumocystis jiroveci* when its classified status shifted from that of a parasite to that of a fungal pathogen.

Microsporidia are organisms that must always live inside other cells, and they have been discovered in a wide variety of species, particularly invertebrates. They are most often seen in worms. The width may vary from 1.5 to 5 μm, and the length can be anywhere from 2 to 7 μm. Unfortunately, the organisms that are discovered in people are often fairly tiny, with lengths ranging from 1.5 to 2 μm. Only recently has more emphasis been placed on the organisms that cause human diseases; before this, awareness and comprehension of human infections were rather limited. This change was triggered as a result of greater knowledge about AIDS in immunocompromised populations. The spores of these organisms possess a polar tubule, it acts as a device for outward protrusion for delivering infectious spore content into cells of the host organism. One of the qualities that separates these animals apart from others is their ability to do this. To this day, seven genera have been identified as causing disease in humans. These include the most frequent *Enterocytozoon* and *Encephalitozoon*, as well as the lesser typical *Pleistophora*, *Brachiola*, *Vittaforma*, *Trachipleistophora*, and "*Microsporidium*," which is a general term for organisms that have not yet been defined. The size of the spores, the arrangement of the nuclei within the spores and growing forms, the total amount of polar tubule coils that are included within the spores, and the interaction between the host cell and the organism are all factors that are used for classification.

Several hundred people with persistent diarrhea have been documented around the world, and microsporidiosis is a serious opportunist disease that may occur in people who are HIV-positive. Cases infected with *Cryptosporidium* spp. could also have numerous illnesses of microsporidia at the same time, and the percentage of such patients could be close to 30%. These results highlight how important it is to consider these species as possible pathogens that can cause diarrhea in individuals who have impaired immune systems, especially those with HIV. On the other hand, due to the fact that antiretroviral combination treatment is now being used, the same reduction in cryptosporidiosis that was shown also in this patient population was also noticed with microsporidiosis. *Microsporidia* is another potential illness-causing agent in people who have had organ transplants, as well as travelers, people who use contact lenses, and elderly people (Pozio et al., 2004).

Lyfe Cycle and Morphology

The phase of the infection that is contagious life cycle is the spore, which would also be the only stage of the life cycle that can survive outside of the host cell. Ingestion is the typical method by which the spore is transferred to a new host; nevertheless, researchers have discovered additional channels of transmission.

The infective sporoplasm must first enter the host cell through the polar tubule in order for infection to take place. The microsporidia reproduce widely inside the cytoplasm of the host cell; the life cycle consists of repetitive divisions that may be binary (merogony) or numerous (schizogony). There is the potential for both merogony and sporogony to take place concurrently within the same cell.

Disease

The first species, *Encephalitozoon cuniculi*, was identified from human diseases in the central nervous system, while the second species, *E.hellem*, was isolated from human eye infections. The first patient was a Japanese child who was nine years old and had neurological manifestations including vomiting, convulsions, fever, headaches, and spells of drowsiness with this condition. This patient was the first person diagnosed with the disease. The spores were extracted from the cerebral fluid and the urine of the patient. This patient in particular responded well to treatment with sulfisoxazole and made a full recovery. In a second instance of *A.cuniculi* infection, the spores were isolated from the urine of a child who was 2 years old who suffered a neurological condition comparable to the first.

Diagnosis

Recovery and identification of microsporidia in clinical specimens can be accomplished using a variety of different methods. Even though the organisms have been recognized in standard histological preparations, it is uncommon for them to stain in a predictable manner; if they stain at all with sections that have been routinely fixed with formalin, paraffin-embedded, and stained with hematoxylin and eosin (HE), the spores might sometimes take on the appearance of gold that is refractory. There is a possibility that the use of formalin contributed to the difficulties; other fixatives are now being researched and tested. When working with the silver stains, acid-fast stains, or PAS stains, it is sometimes possible to see the spores extremely clearly. It has also been discovered that modified Gram stains are sensitive, despite the fact that they are not usually standardized. The spore has a tiny posterior body that is positive for PAS, silver may be seen on the surface of the spore coat, and it is resistant to the acid of the spores may be varied. Methods such as antigen detection, molecular analysis, and serological testing are further examples of diagnostic procedures.

Treatment

Although quite a few medications have been tested, the results have been somewhat inconsistent. Agents such as lomotil, metronidazole, octreotide, itraconazole, primaquine, loperamide, albendazole, and sulfosalazine have been utilized in diverse individuals.

Malaria spp.

Plasmodium parasites continue to be responsible for more deaths than any other infectious germs, despite malaria being one of the oldest human diseases for which there is historical evidence. In humans, the two species *Plasmodium vivax* and *Plasmodium falciparum* are responsible for the majority of infections; the others are *P.ovale* and *P.malariae.*

Life Cycle and Morphology

The female anopheline mosquito is responsible for transmitting the malaria parasite. During the process of the vector feeding on a blood meal, the sporozoites that are stored in the salivary glands of the mosquito are released to the site of the puncture. In an hour, these infectious phases arrive in the liver after traveling through the bloodstream. Once there, they invade hepatocytes and start growing, which marks the beginning of the pre-erythrocytic cycle, also known as the main exoerythrocytic cycle. The sporozoites undergo a rounding and ovalization process and then begin to divide repeatedly. The result of this schizogony is a significant increase in the number of exoerythrocytic merozoites. After leaving the liver, these merozoites initiate the erythrocytic cycle by invading red blood cells (RBCs), marking the beginning of the process.

After the red blood cells and reticulocytes have been taken over by the parasites, the latter continue to proliferate and sustain themselves on the hemoglobin. The merozoite has vacuoles, is ring-shaped, resembles amoebae to a certain extent, and lacks nuclei when it is contained inside the RBC. The nucleus starts to split, and the trophozoite that is evolving into a schizont is termed that. The adult schizont has merozoites inside it, and these merozoites are then discharged into the circulation. However, some merozoites can infect RBCs, resulting in the beginning of a new cycle of erythrocytic schizogony. The immune system is able to destroy a significant number of merozoites.

Disease

The patient does not show any symptoms from the moment they were bitten by the mosquito until at least a week after the bite. The liver is the location where the organisms are replicating themselves throughout this time period. Malaria may cause a variety of clinical signs, including anemia, splenomegaly, and the characteristic paroxysm, which is characterized by a cold stage, fever, and sweats. Malaria has the ability to mimic the signs and symptoms of a great many different diseases, including gastroenteritis, pneumonia, meningitis, encephalitis, and hepatitis.

Diagnosis

Patients who have a history of traveling in a region where malaria is prevalent are often considered to be at a higher risk of developing the disease. Although the Giemsa stain is the one that is suggested for all parasite blood tests, other blood stains, such as the Wrights' stain, are also capable of revealing the parasitic organisms. It is permissible to use blood that has been obtained using the EDTA anticoagulant. Additionally, when taking anticoagulants, it should always be kept in mind that maintaining the proper proportions of blood to anticoagulant is critical for the morphology of a healthy body. This ratio is crucial to keep in mind. Heparin is another option, although EDTA is recommended.

It is suggested to get blood through a finger stick, especially when the amount of blood needed is quite small. There is often a correlation between the density of known polymorphonuclear leukocyte parasites and the severity of the disease. The presence of pigmented neutrophils (also called monocytes) has been associated with cerebral malaria, as well as death in infants suffering from severe malaria.

P.vivax, often known as benign Tertian malaria, has a cycle of 48 hours and has a propensity to infect young cells. Schuffner's spots and enlarged RBCs are usual findings in smears. Additionally, a tiny ring and a trophozoite that is highly ameboid may be detected. The mature schizont includes 12-24 merozoites.

P.ovale also has a cycle of 48 hours, and it has a propensity to infect both young and old cells. In comparison to *P.vivax*, it has a ring that is less thick, and its trophozoite is less ameboid in appearance. A developed schizont will have a total of eight merozoites.

P. malariae, which causes quartan malaria, has a cycle of 72 hours (due to its long incubation time), and it has a propensity to infect older cells. The mature schizont includes 6-12 merozoites.

P. falciparum is the parasite responsible for the most severe form of malaria (malignant tertian malaria) and has a cycle that lasts between 36 and 48 hours. Because it has a propensity to infect any cell, regardless of its age, this may lead to a high-force infection. It possesses gametocytes that are formed like a crescent.

Malaria is one of the few parasite diseases regarded as an urgent risk to a person's life. Patients who have received the diagnosis of *P. falciparum* malaria should be treated as if they are experiencing a medical emergency since the disease may quickly lead to death. Malaria is one of the very few parasite diseases that may pose an immediate danger to a person's life. For a significant amount of time, thin or thick blood films that have been stained with Giemsa and regarded as the "gold standard" for diagnosing malaria have been utilized.

Treatment

Over the last several years, malaria has become a more widespread health concern. Both the growth in *P. falciparum*'s resistance to a wide number of medications and the progress that has been made in the treatment of severe disease complications have contributed to the complexity that has been introduced into therapy. The stages of malaria that a treatment is effective against are used to categorize different types of antimalarial medication. These medications are often referred to as tissue schizonticides, blood schizonticides, gametocytocidal, and sporonticides. Tissue schizonticides are responsible for the death of tissue schizonts, while blood schizonticides are responsible for the death of blood schizonts. Gametocytocides destroy gametocytes. Sporonticides inhibit the production of sporozoites within the mosquito.

Toxoplasma Gondii

Toxoplasma gondii is found all over the world, it is closely linked to other types of coccidiosis, and it also has certain characteristics with the parasites that cause malaria. T.gondii is capable of infecting a wide variety of animals in addition to humans; nevertheless, the domestic cat as well as different species belonging to the family Felidae are the parasite's definitive hosts.

Life Cycle and Morphology

It is possible for humans to get the virus in a few different ways. One of these ways is by the unintentional intake of oocysts that have been shed in cat feces. Another method is through the consumption of foods that are served rare or uncooked, especially lamb, pig, or deer. Additionally, transmission may occur when a person is still in the womb, through blood transfusions, or even during organ transplants. After receiving a liver transplant, toxoplasmosis should be taken into consideration as a potential cause of the failure of multiple organs. Consumption of rare or raw meat is probably the most prevalent route of transmission of this disease. Cat feces include oocysts that range in size from 9 to 11 μm in width and 11 to 14 μm in length. These oocysts have two sporocysts inside them, and each sporocyst has four sporozoites inside it. After being exposed to any one of the three infectious stages through ingestion of *T.gondii*, which are tachyzoites grouped together, bradyzoites contained inside tissue cysts, or sporozoites contained within oocysts, cats will produce oocysts that they will then shed. Birds, tiny rodents, and other sources of raw meat may transmit disease to cats when consumed by them. During the tachyzoite-induced phase during the course of the life cycle of Toxoplasma gondii in cats, the animals can produce up to 360 million oocysts per day and will continue to do so for a period of between four and six days. Cats can continue to shed oocysts as long as they remain infected (Dubey, 2002).

The tachyzoites, bradyzoites, and sporozoites are the three phases of the *T.gondii* life cycle that are infectious to humans. Tachyzoites are able to quickly reproduce somewhere inside the cells of the intermediary host. This encompasses people as well as a wide variety of other species, as well as in the nonintestinal epithelial cells of the definitive host, which includes cats. The tissue cysts contain bradyzoites, which reproduce extremely slowly and may include anything from a few to hundreds of organisms. The intramuscular cysts can grow to be as large as 100 millimeters in diameter. Although the tissue cysts have the potential to develop in visceral organs such as the kidneys, liver, and lungs; nevertheless, they are more often seen in neuromuscular tissues such as the eyes and brain, as well as in cardiac and skeletal muscle. This is because these tissues are more prone to the development of cysts. The presence of an intact tissue cyst does not trigger an inflammatory response and may continue for the host's entire life.

Both of these organisms are classified as obligatory intracellular parasites that may manifest themselves in two distinct ways inside the human host. During the early and more severe stages of the infection, it is common to see trophozoites or tachyzoites that are actively growing. The resting forms, also known as cysts, are most often seen in the brain and muscle, most likely as a consequence of an immunological response from the host. The trophozoites and bradyzoites, which develop more slowly, are contained inside the cysts. Giemsa is the most often used stain; it gives a light blue color to the cytoplasm and a red color to the nucleus. Chronic infections are responsible for the formation of the cysts, and the organisms that reside inside the wall of the cyst are highly periodic acid-Schiff positive. During the acute phase, there might be clusters of tachyzoites that have the appearance of cysts; nevertheless, they are not strongly positive for periodic acid-Schiff and have been given the name pseudocysts.

Disease

Congenital toxoplasmosis, acquired toxoplasmosis, acquired or reactivated toxoplasmosis in immunosuppressed or immunodeficient individuals, ocular toxoplasmosis, and acquired toxoplasmosis are the four subtypes of toxoplasmosis that may be distinguished. Before the development of highly active antiretroviral medications, people with AIDS were known to have a higher risk of contracting the opportunistic disease "toxoplasma encephalitis," which may result in death. If treatment is not received, this condition is lethal. Although the vast majority of AIDS patients with toxoplasma encephalitis have detectable IgG antibodies to *T.gondii*, it is possible that less than 5% of these individuals do not have antibodies in their blood. *T.gondii* may also present itself psychologically in immunocompromised people living with AIDS, particularly those people whose dormant infections have become active again. Delusions, auditory hallucinations, and cognitive disorders are some of the symptoms that can accompany an altered mental state, which affects around 60% of patients. Infections that are present at birth are called congenital infections, and they are caused by the transmission of parasites from a mother to her unborn child whenever the mother suffers from a primary infection when she is pregnant, and the parasites are carried in the mother's blood. During the acute phase of infection, there are no clinical signs are observed in 0% of patients. If the woman contracts the virus during her first or second trimester of pregnancy, the infection may be passed on to the fetus and cause very severe congenital symptoms. Inflammation of the retina, calcification of the brain, and other related conditions on occasion, hydrocephalus or microcephaly are some of the symptoms that might happen in these babies shortly after delivery or shortly after birth itself.

Diagnosis

Mostly referred to as a diagnosis is reached by a series of serologic investigations. The polymerase chain reaction (PCR), some of the other procedures, include the analysis of a biopsy sample, buffy coat cells, or cerebrospinal fluid, as well as the isolation of the microorganism in tissue culture or in animal models. The Sabin-Feldman dye test was one of the first tests that were used to diagnose toxoplasmosis. The test was based on the observation that *T.*gondii is in the presence of immune serum, reducing its receptivity to the methylene blue dye that it normally uses.

Treatment

Sulfonamides and pyrimethamine are examples of medications that have been shown to be useful, either alone or in combination with other medicines. In select situations, clindamycin and spiramycin have also been used as treatment options.

Conclusion

In recent years, with the development of diagnostic possibilities and the discovery of new methods, the possibility of a more precise and early diagnosis has arisen. This is despite the fact that infections caused by parasites, which are an important part of microbiology, in the central nervous system are known to be quite complex and difficult to recognize diseases.

References

Alejandre-Aguilar, R., Calvo-Méndez, M. L., Nogueda-Torres, B., & de la Jara-Alcocer, F. (1998). Maintenance of Acanthamoeba culbertsoni by cryopreservation. *Journal of Parasitology, 84*(5), 1261-1264. *https://doi.org/10.2307/3284685.*

Axelsson-Olsson, D., Waldenstrom, J., Broman, T., Olsen, B., & Holmberg, M. (2005). Protozoan Acanthamoeba polyphaga as a potential reservoir for Campylobacter jejuni. *Applied Environmental Microbiology, 71*(2), 987-992. *https://doi.org/10.1128/AEM.71.2.987-992.2005.*

Beattie, T. K., Seal, D. V., Tomlinson, A. K., McFadyen, A. K., & Grimason, A. M. (2003). Determination of amoebicidal activities of multipurpose contact lens solutions by using a most probable number enumeration technique. *Journal of Clinical Microbiology, 41*(7), 2992-3000. *https://doi.org/10.1128/JCM.41.7.2992-3000.2003.*

Booton, G. C., Carmichael, J. R., Visvesvara, G. S., Byers, T. J., & Fuerst, P. A. (2003a). Genotyping of Balamuthia mandrillaris based on nuclear 18S and mitochondrial 16S rRNA genes. *American Journal of Tropical Medicine and Hygiene, 68*(1), 65-69. *https://doi.org/10.4269/ajtmh.2003.68.65.*

Booton, G. C., Carmichael, J. R., Visvesvara, G. S., Byers, T. J., & Fuerst, P. A. (2003b). Identification of Balamuthia mandrillaris by PCR assay using the mitochondrial 16S rRNA gene as a target. *Journal of Clinical Microbiology, 41*(1), 453-455. *https://doi.org/10.1128/JCM.41.1.453-455.2003.*

Dubey, J. P. (2002). The tachyzoite-induced life cycle of Toxoplasma gondii in cats. *Journal of Parasitology, 88*(4), 713-717. *https://doi.org/10.1645/0022-3395(2002)088[0713:TILCOT]2.0.CO;2.*

Garcia, S. L. (2007). *Diagnostic Medical Parasitology, Fifth Edition.* ASM Press, Washington, D.C., 102-122.

Grace, E., Asbill, S., & Virga, K. (2015). *Antimicrobial Agents and Chemotherapy, 59*(11), 6677-6681. *https://doi.org/10.1128/AAC.01293-15.*

Gelman, B. B., Popov, V., Chaljub, G., Nader, R., Rauf, S. J., Nauta, H. W., & Visvesvara, G. S. (2003). Neuropathological and ultrastructural features of amebic encephalitis caused by Sappinia diploidea. *Journal of Neuropathology and Experimental Neurology, 62*(10), 990-998. *https://doi.org/10.1093/jnen/62.10.990.*

Greub, G., & Raoult, D. (2004). Microorganisms resistant to free-living amoebae. *Clinical Microbiological Reviews, 17*(2), 413-443. *https://doi.org/10.1128/CMR.17.2.413-433.2004.*

Güeméz, A., & Garcia, E. (2021). Primary amoebic meningoencephalitis by Naegleria fowleri: Pathogenesis and treatment. *Biomolecules, 11*, 1320-1323. *https://doi.org/10.3390/biom11091320.*

Jayasekera, S. J., Sissons, J., Tucker, J., Rogers, C., Nolder, D., Warhurst, D., Alsan, S., White, J. M., Higgins, E. M., & Khan, N. A. (2004). Post-mortem culture of Balamuthia mandrillaris from the brain and cerebrospinal fluid of a case of granulomatous amoebic meningoencephalitis using human brain microvascular endothelial cells. *Journal of Medical Microbiology, 53*(10), 1007-1012. *https://doi.org/10.1099/jmm.0.45721-0.*

Kilvington, S., Gray, T., Dart, J., Morlet, N., Beeching, J. R., Frazer, D. G., & Matheson, M. (2004). Acanthamoeba keratitis: The role of domestic tap water contamination in the United Kingdom. *Investigative Ophthalmology and Visual Science, 45*(1), 165-169. *https://doi.org/10.1167/iovs.03-0559.*

Kinnear, F. B. (2003). Cytopathogenicity of Acanthamoeba, Vahlkampfia, and Hartmanella: Quantitative and qualitative in vitro studies on keratocytes. *Journal of Infection, 46*(4), 228-237. *https://doi.org/10.1053/jinf.2002.1116.*

Kum, S. J., Lee, H. W., Jung, H. R., Choe, M., & Kim, S. P. (2019). Amoebic encephalitis caused by Balamuthia mandrillaris. *Journal of Pathology and Translational Medicine, 53*(5), 327-331. *https://doi.org/10.4132/jptm.2019.05.14.*

Mansfield, L. S., & Jenkins, A. A. (2004). Cyclospora cayetanensis, a food- and waterborne coccidian parasite. *Veterinary Parasitology, 126*(1-2), 73-90. *https://doi.org/10.1016/j.vetpar.2004.09.011.*

Marciano-Cabral, F., & Cabral, G. (2003). Acanthamoeba spp. as agents of disease in humans. *Clinical Microbiology Reviews, 16*(2), 273-307. *https://doi.org/10.1128/CMR.16.2.273-307.2003.*

McBride, J., Ingram, P. R., Henriquez, F. L., & Roberts, C. W. (2005). Development of colorimetric microtiter plate assay for assessment of antimicrobials against Acanthamoeba. *Journal of Clinical Microbiology, 43*(2), 629-634. *https://doi.org/10.1128/JCM.43.2.629-634.2005.*

Pasricha, G., Sharma, S., Garg, P., & Aggarwal, R. K. (2003). Use of 18S rRNA gene-based PCR assay for diagnosis of Acanthamoeba keratitis in non-contact lens wearers in India. *Journal of Clinical Microbiology, 41*(7), 3206-3211. *https://doi.org/10.1128/JCM.41.7.3206-3211.2003.*

Pozio, E., Rivasi, F., & Caccio, S. M. (2004). Infection with Cryptosporidium hominis and reinfection with Cryptosporidium parvum in transplanted ileum. *APMIS, 112*(5), 309-313. *https://doi.org/10.1111/j.1600-0463.2004.apm11204-0513.x.*

Schuster, F. L. (2002). Cultivation of pathogenic and opportunistic free-living amebas. *Clinical Microbiology Reviews, 15*(3), 342-354. *https://doi.org/10.1128/CMR.15.3.342-354.2002.*

Schuster, F. L., Dunnebacke, T. H., Booton, G. C., Yagi, S., Kohnmeier, C. K., Glaser, C., Vugia, D., Bakardjiev, A., Azimi, P., Maddux-Gonzalez, M., & Visvesvara, G. S. (2003). Environmental isolation of Balamuthia mandrillaris associated with a case of amebic encephalitis. *Journal of Clinical Microbiology, 41*(7), 3175-3180. *https://doi.org/10.1128/JCM.41.7.3175-3180.2003.*

Schuster, F. L., & Visvesvara, G. S. (2004a). Free-living amoebae as opportunistic and non-opportunistic pathogens of humans and animals. *International Journal of Parasitology, 34*(9), 1001-1027. *https://doi.org/10.1016/j.ijpara.2004.06.004.*

Schuster, F. L., & Visvesvara, G. S. (2004b). Opportunistic amoebae: Challenges in prophylaxis and treatment. *Drug Resistance Update, 7*(1-2), 41-51. *https://doi.org/10.1016/j.drup.2004.01.002.*

Siddiqui, R., Mungroo, M. R., Anuar, T. S., Alharbi, A. M., Alfahemi, H., Elmoselhi, A. B., & Khan, N. A. (2022). Antiamoebic properties of laboratory and clinically used drugs against Naegleria fowleri and Balamuthia mandrillaris. *Antibiotics, 11. https://doi.org/10.3390/antibiotics11060749.*

Thomas, V., Bouchez, T., Nicolas, V., Robert, S., Loret, J. F., & Levi, Y. (2004). Amoebae in domestic water systems: Resistance to disinfection treatments and implication in Legionella persistence. *Journal of Applied Microbiology, 97*(5), 950-963. *https://doi.org/10.1111/j.1365-2672.2004.02391.x.*

Visvesvara, G. S., Moura, H., & Schuster, Frederick. (2007). Pathogenic and opportunistic free-living amoebae: Acanthamoeba spp., Balamuthia mandrillaris, Naegleria fowleri and Sappinia diploidea. *FEMS Immunology and Medical Microbiology, 50*(1), 1-26. *https://doi.org/10.1111/j.1574-695X.2007.00232.x.*

Chapter 14

HIV and the Central Nervous System

Meltem Karslıoğlu*, **MD**
Department of Infectious Disease and Clinical Microbiology,
Samsun Gazi State Hospital, Samsun, Turkiye

Abstract

HIV (Human Immune Deficiency Virus) infection becomes increasingly widespread. The central nervous system takes a significant place in this infection, which can affect all systems. In addition to HIV-related clinical manifestations, opportunistic pathogens, malignancies, and multiple drug use due to immunodeficiency also contribute to neurocognitive disorders. It is crucial to know these diseases to reduce morbidity and mortality. HIV-associated neurocognitive disorder (HAND) is also observed in cases administered antiretroviral therapy (ART). The prevalence of opportunistic pathogens has decreased significantly with the widespread use of ART.

Keywords: HIV, central nervous system, HIV-associated ensephalopathy

Introduction

Changes in memory, concentration, attention, and motor skills are common in patients with HIV/AIDS (Shapshak et al., 2011). Since various disorders can cause these symptoms, an accurate diagnosis is essential for treatment planning (Price, 1996). When there is no alternative cause other than HIV infection, such disorders are collectively classified as HIV-associated

* Corresponding Author's Email: celikmltm@hotmail.com.

In: Central Nervous System Infections
Editor: Mustafa Usanmaz
ISBN: 979-8-89113-660-1

neurocognitive disorders (HAND) (Shapshak et al., 2011; Price, 1996; Antinori et al., 2007).

Neurocognitive deficits developing in individuals with HIV/AIDS and not having an alternative explanation other than HIV infection were first classified in 2007 as the "Frascati criteria" by the HIV Neurobehavioral Research Center at the University of California, San Diego (Antinori et al., 2007);

Asymptomatic neurocognitive impairment (ANI) – It is defined as one standard deviation or being below the average in at least two cognitive domains on standard neuropsychological tests without symptomatic or observable functional impairment.

Mild neurocognitive disorder (MND) – It is defined as a standard deviation or being below the average in at least two cognitive domains, along with mild symptomatic or functional impairment on standard neuropsychological tests.

HIV-associated dementia (HAD) – It is defined as an impairment in activities of daily living and two standard deviations or being below the average in at least two cognitive domains on standard neuropsychological tests.

Pathophysiology

HIV spreads to the central nervous system (CNS) on the first days of systemic infection and can be detected in the cerebrospinal fluid (CSF) in most untreated patients (McCutchan et al., 2007). https://www.uptodate.com/contents/hiv-associated-neurocognitive-disorders-epidemiology-clinical-manifestations-and-diagnosis/abstract/6.

In the beginning, viruses detected in the CSF are the same as those detected in the blood but later change their character. Whereas viruses detected in the blood show T lymphocyte tropism, viruses detected in the CSF change to macrophage-tropic (M-tropic). It is unclear whether M-tropic viruses originate from the CNS or infected monocytes (González-Scarano & Martín-García, 2005).

Although antiretroviral therapy (ART) reduces HIV RNA in the CSF, immune activation is detected in the CNS even after persistent viral suppression in a significant part of patients (Edén et al., 2007). The widespread use of antiretroviral therapy (ART) has been associated with a significant decrease in the incidence of severe neurocognitive impairment (d'Arminio Monforte et al., 2004).

The CASCADE cohort showed that the incidence of HAD decreased from 6.49 to 0.66 per year compared to the pre-ART period in 15,380 patients with HIV/AIDS followed up between 2003 and 2006 (Bhaskaran et al., 2008). https://www.uptodate.com/contents/hiv-associated-neurocognitive-disorders-epidemiology-clinical-manifestations-and-diagnosis/abstract/29.

Risk Factors

HIV-Related Factors

A few studies have associated low CD4 cell count with neurocognitive impairment (Valcour et al., 2006). The CASCADE study determined low CD4 cell count, advanced age, duration of HIV infection, and the presence of AIDS-defining disease as risk factors for HAD development (Bhaskaran et al., 2008). Immunosuppression due to HIV infection and the associated viral replication continuing in the CNS may initiate a neuropathic process even after treatment and CD4 cell increase (Dunfee et al., 2006).

Comorbidities

There is a higher prevalence of neurocognitive deficits and dementia in HIV patients older than 50 than in younger patients (Cherner et al., 2004). A 12-year study conducted on HIV patients showed that comorbidities such as advanced age, diabetes, hypertension, chronic lung disease, depression, and a history of cannabis use contributed to the decrease in cognitive status (Heaton et al., 2022).

Anemia, vascular diseases, and metabolic syndrome are other associated comorbidities in the elderly (McCutchan et al., 2012). Although traditional cardiovascular risk factors are associated with the risk of developing dementia in the general population and HIV patients, HIV-related factors such as CD4 cell count or viral load are more associated with neurocognitive disorders .

Hepatitis C virus (HCV) can pass to the CNS through macrophages and infect microglia and astrocytes. The HCV core protein can cause neuronal damage through the production of proinflammatory cytokines. Therefore, it has been associated with neurocognitive disorders in coinfected patients. Previous toxoplasma infection has also been found to be associated with neurocognitive disorders (Moulignier & Costagliola, 2021, Laskus et al., 2002, Bharti et al., 2016).

Host Genetic Factors

Polymorphisms in many genes, including those encoding apolipoprotein E4, the chemokine receptor CCR2, and monocyte chemoattractant protein-1, have been associated with the presence or development of HAD (Gonzalez et al., 2002).

The Use of Antiretroviral Therapy (ART)

HIV-associated dementia (HAD) typically occurs in patients with advanced, untreated HIV infection, CD4 cell count below 200 cells/microL, and high viral load. Patients undergoing ART are unlikely to have neurocognitive disorders. Nevertheless, although viral load decreases in the plasma of patients using ART regularly, viral RNA can rarely be detected in the CSF, and this condition is called "CNS escape syndrome."

HIV-Associated Dementia (HAD)

It is characterized by subcortical dysfunction, impaired concentration, psychomotor impairment, and depressive symptoms and predominantly occurs in patients with untreated HIV infection. Typically, cognitive dysfunction is evident and markedly impairs functional status. Patients with HAD are usually very slow and forgetful in their daily activities and may become lost while walking or driving.

The absence of higher cortical dysfunctions, including aphasia, agnosia, and apraxia, helps to distinguish HAD from classical "cortical" dementia, such as Alzheimer's disease. Patients usually have apathy and lack of motivation (abulia) (Grill & Price, 2014). They may also experience anxiety, insomnia, restlessness, and weight loss. However, crying spells are distinguished from depression by the absence of pronounced sadness. Cerebral atrophy is evident on brain imaging in HAD patients (Schouten et al., 2011, Dal Pan et al., 1992). It mainly impacts the basal ganglia (particularly the caudate), white matter, and cortical regions. More advanced neuroimaging techniques such as magnetic resonance spectroscopy, functional MRI, and positron emission tomography (PET) show abnormalities in subcortical regions even in patients with milder neurocognitive impairments (Roc et al., 2007).

CSF protein is often high in HAD patients not undergoing ART. These findings are not specific to HAD patients and can be observed in many untreated HIV patients without neurocognitive disorders. The HIV RNA level from the CSF does not provide diagnostic benefits.

CNS Viral Escape Syndrome

In patients presenting with neurological deficits and not receiving ART, demonstrating HIV replication in the CSF despite low HIV RNA levels was defined as "CNS viral escape syndrome" (Peluso et al., 2012). HIV RNA was determined at a detectable level in the CSF in 7.1% of patients who were followed up for an average of 30 months and achieved viral suppression with ART (Edén et al., 2010).

Immune Reconstitution Inflammatory Syndrome (IRIS)

Severe new-onset neurological symptoms may rarely occur due to HIV-associated immune reconstitution inflammatory syndrome (IRIS). This condition may present as severe CD8 cell-derived encephalitis with diffuse white and gray matter abnormalities on MRI and CD8 cell pleocytosis in the CSF (Lescure et al., 2013).

Diagnosis

The diagnosis is established in an HIV patient with a neurocognitive disorder (especially if it is new or predicted to progress) by a history, physical examination, and neuropsychological tests. HIV-associated dementia (HAD), minor neurocognitive disorder (MND), or asymptomatic neurocognitive impairment (ANI) can only be classified by the application of neuropsychological tests by experts.

Differential Diagnosis

Cognitive impairment in HIV patients may be a symptom of numerous other disease processes. The differential diagnosis depends on the degree of immunosuppression and whether the patient takes antiretroviral agents.

Central Nervous System (CNS) Infections

Toxoplasma

Toxoplasmosis is caused by an intracellular protozoan agent named *Toxoplasma gondii*. It is the most common central nervous system infection in patients with acquired immunodeficiency who do not receive appropriate prophylaxis. In these patients, the parasite, which is usually latent, can be activated when the CD4 count decreases below 100 cells/microL (Porter & Sande, 1992, San-Andrés et al., 2003, Renold et al., 1992, Luft & Remington, 1992). The central nervous system is the most common site of reactivation. Transmission in humans usually occurs by the ingestion of oocysts from cat feces, contaminated soil, cat litter, and/or undercooked meat of infected animals. Oocysts spread from the intestinal epithelium to the entire body. They may remain in the form of cysts in tissues lifelong. After effective antiretroviral therapy (ART) has started to be used, the incidence of toxoplasma-induced encephalitis (TE) has decreased in HIV-positive patients. For example, the number of annual hospitalizations for toxoplasmosis among HIV patients in the United States of America has decreased from over 10,000 in 1995 to 2985 in 2008 (jones & Roberts,2008). Headache, fever, and changes in consciousness are usually observed in patients. Neurological disorders are caused by increased intracranial pressure. Patients may present with epileptic seizures. Focal neurological deficits may also accompany them. Stupor and coma may also be observed (Porter & Sande, 1992).

There are no routine laboratory findings specific to toxoplasmosis. Mononuclear pleocytosis may be present in the cerebrospinal fluid (CSF) (Andrews & Kenefick, 1993). Toxoplasma IgG antibodies are positive in most patients with toxoplasma encephalitis (TE). However, their being negative does not exclude the diagnosis of TE (National Institutes of Health, 2023). PCR should be sent from the CSF by performing a lumbar puncture. Thus, differential diagnosis can also be made for infectious and non-infectious causes. If the clinical suspicion of PCR negativity is high, it does not exclude

also be observed in patients with normal cell counts (Aksamit, 2012). However, the incidence of PML has decreased after the widespread use of ART (Sacktor, 2002). Patients usually present with symptoms such as hemiparesis, dementia, speech, vision, and gait disturbances. Fever and headaches do not occur very frequently. If there is a clinical suspicion of PML and compatible imaging in HIV-infected patients, lumbar puncture should be carried out, especially for sending JCV PCR. The leukocyte count in the CSF is <20 cells/microL. The protein level is usually lower than 100 mg/dL, and a mild protein increase can be observed. With the recovery of the host immunity in HIV patients receiving treatment, the cell count may increase above 20 cells/microL; otherwise, a different infectious cause must be considered (Aksamit, 2012).

PML diagnosis is established by demonstrating JCV PCR in the CSF. In addition to JCV PCR, routine examinations of the CSF for differential diagnosis, cytology, and flow cytometry (to exclude lymphoma) should be carried out, and PCR should be sent for cryptococcal antigen and Epstein-Barr virus, varicella-zoster virus, cytomegalovirus, and herpes simplex virus-1 and 2. In case a lumbar puncture does not support the diagnosis, alternative diagnoses should be reviewed, and a repeat lumbar puncture should be considered. A brain biopsy must be performed for a differential and definitive diagnosis. The typical histopathological triad of PML (demyelination, dysmorphic astrocytes, and enlarged oligodendroglial nuclei) is not seen in other neurological disorders (Berger et al., 2013).

In patients having a CD4 count of 50-100 cells/microL, focal/multifocal white matter lesions not typically causing a mass effect can be observed on brain MRI, along with the above-mentioned neurological complaints. Lesions typically do not enhance contrast, and hemorrhage is not observed.

Primary central nervous system (CNS) lymphoma can also mimic PML lesions. Nevertheless, there is extensive contrast involvement in imaging, and cytology from the CSF and EBV PCR may be helpful in the differential diagnosis.

CNS Malignancies

Primary Central Nervous System Lymphoma

HIV-associated infections predispose individuals to the development of some cancers. Kaposi's sarcoma, non-Hodgkin's lymphoma (NHL), primary central nervous system lymphoma (PCNSL), and invasive cervical carcinoma are among the AIDS-defining diseases.

PCNSL accounts for approximately 10-15 percent of non-Hodgkin's lymphomas (NHL) in HIV-infected individuals (Coté et al., 1997). Diffuse large B-cell lymphoma is the most common histology (Raez et al., 1998).

PCNSL represents the second CNS localized lesion after toxoplasmosis in HIV/AIDS patients. Its pathogenesis is related to EBV infection. A decrease in the count of EBV-specific CD4+ T cells and the development of loss of function are the main causes of the present clinical manifestation. It is usually observed in patients with CD4 count below 50 cells/microL (Raez et al., 1998, Moulignier et al., 2017).

Low CD4 cell count, high HIV viral load, and hepatitis B and hepatitis C coinfection are poor prognostic factors. The incidence of PCNSL has decreased with the widespread use of ART.

Depending on the location and size of the lesions in the brain, the amount of edema in the surrounding tissues, and the mass effect, it may present with various focal or diffuse neurological signs and symptoms. Patients may present with headache, memory loss, confusion, hemiparesis, aphasia, and epileptic seizures. B symptoms may accompany in 80% of patients (Baumgartner et al., 1990).

If there are no contraindications as a result of imaging, lumbar puncture should be performed, and EBV PCR, JC PCR, flow cytometry, and/or cytology should be sent in addition to routine examinations. It should be remembered that HIV-associated PSSS can be an extremely aggressive neoplasm and delay in diagnosis can lead to devastating consequences. Hence, diagnostic biopsies should be kept in mind immediately after admission. To increase diagnostic yield, pre-biopsy use of glucocorticoids should be avoided (Chappell et al., 1992). It may be sufficient to detect Epstein-Barr virus (EBV) DNA in the CSF for treatment in selected patients who cannot be biopsied and have typical clinical and radiographic findings for PCNSL.

On non-contrast computed tomography (CT), lesions are typically isodense or hyperdense relative to gray matter, and cerebral edema is frequently observed (Antinori et al., 1997, Thurnher et al., 1997). On MRI, there may be a single lesion or multiple lesions of roughly equal size, and they show contrast enhancement (Johnson et al., 1997).

Other Dementia Syndromes

Patients with HIV infection controlled by ART may develop other dementia diseases with longer survival. Alzheimer's disease can usually be differentiated into states of memory loss associated with other "cortical" abnormalities such as aphasia and apraxia.

Nutritional Deficiencies

Cognitive impairment due to vitamin B12 deficiency may be accompanied by other neurological symptoms, such as paresthesias and sensory deficits. Vitamin B12 deficiency can be easily identified by laboratory tests.

Endocrine Disorders

Hormonal abnormalities, such as thyroid dysfunction and adrenal insufficiency, are also frequently observed in HIV infection and may cause cognitive dysfunction.

Use of Banned Substances or Psychiatric Disorder

The use of banned substances is among the risk factors in the diagnosis of HAND, and it may also cause cognitive dysfunction independent of the diagnosis of HAND, like other psychiatric disorders. A detailed anamnesis may help in the differential diagnosis.

Multiple Drug Use

Especially anticholinergic agents, opioids, and anxiolytics may adversely impact cognitive status (Rubin et al., 2018, Cooley et al., 2021). The discontinuation of these drugs may improve the state of consciousness.

Conclusion

The number of patients with HIV/AIDS increases every day, which brings about HIV-related complications. Possible neurological complications should be considered, and a differential diagnosis should be established. First, HIV diagnosis should be established early, and diseases that cause neurocognitive dysfunction by impacting the central nervous system should be evaluated with a multidisciplinary approach.

References

Aksamit, A. J. (2013). Progressive multifocal leukoencephalopathy. In *Viral Infections of the Human Nervous System* (pp. 65-86). Springer. https://doi.org/10.1007/978-3-0348-0425-7_4.

Altınkaya, A. (2014). *Nörosifiliz Hastalarının Klinik Özellikleri [Clinical Features of Patients With Neuroshyphilis]* (Master Thesis). İstanbul Bilim University, Faculty of Medicine, İstanbul.

Andrews, B. T., & Kenefick, T. P. (1993). Neurosurgical management of the acquired immunodeficiency syndrome: An update. *Western Journal of Medicine, 158*(3), 249.

Antinori, A., Ammassari, A., De Luca, A., Cingolani, A., Murri, R., Scoppettuolo, G., Fortini, M., Tartaglione, T., Larocca, L. M., Zannoni, G., Cattani, P., Grillo, R., Roselli, R., Iacoangeli, M., Scerrati, M., & Ortona, L. (1997). Diagnosis of AIDS-related focal brain lesions: A decision-making analysis based on clinical and neuroradiologic characteristics combined with polymerase chain reaction assays in CSF. *Neurology, 48*(3), 687-694. https://doi.org/10.1212/WNL.48.3.687.

Antinori, A., Arendt, G., Becker, J. T., Brew, B. J., Byrd, D. A., Cherner, M., Clifford, D. B., Cinque, P., Epstein, L. G., Goodkin, K., Gisslen, M., Grant, I., Heaton, R. K., Joseph, J., Marder, K., Marra, C. M., McArthur, J. C., Nunn, M., Price, R. W., Pulliam, L., Robertson, K. R., Sacktor, N., Valcour, V., & Wojna, V. E. (2007). Updated research nosology for HIV-associated neurocognitive disorders. *Neurology, 69*(18), 1789-1799. https://doi.org/10.1212/01.WNL.0000287431.88658.8b.

Arribas, J. R., Storch, G. A., Clifford, D. B., & Tselis, A. C. (1996). Cytomegalovirus encephalitis. *Annals of Internal Medicine, 125*(7), 577-587. https://doi.org/10.7326/0003-4819-125-7-199610010-00008.

Arribas, J. R., Clifford, D. B., Fichtenbaum, C. J., Commins, D. L., Powderly, W. G., & Storch, G. A. (1995). Level of cytomegalovirus (CMV) DNA in cerebrospinal fluid of subjects with AIDS and CMV infection of the central nervous system. *Journal of Infectious Diseases, 172*(2), 527-531. https://doi.org/10.1093/infdis/172.2.527.

Bamba, S., Lortholary, O., Sawadogo, A., Millogo, A., Guiguemdé, R. T., & Bretagne, S. (2012). Decreasing incidence of cryptococcal meningitis in West Africa in the era of highly active antiretroviral therapy. *AIDS, 26*(8), 1039-1041. https://doi.org/10.1097/QAD.0b013e328352d1d8.

Berger, J. R., Aksamit, A. J., Clifford, D. B., Davis, L., Koralnik, I. J., Sejvar, J. J., Bartt, R., Major, E. O., & Nath, A. (2013). PML diagnostic criteria: Consensus statement from the AAN Neuroinfectious Disease Section. *Neurology, 80*(15), 1430-1438. https://doi.org/10.1212/WNL.0b013e31828c2fa1.

Bharti, A. R., McCutchan, A., Deutsch, R., Smith, D. M., Ellis, R. J., Cherner, M., Woods, S. P., Heaton, R. K., Grant, I., & Letendre, S. L. (2016). Latent toxoplasma infection and higher toxoplasma gondii immunoglobulin G levels are associated with worse neurocognitive functioning in HIV-infected adults. *Clinical Infectious Diseases.* https://doi.org/10.1093/cid/ciw655.

Bhaskaran, K., Mussini, C., Antinori, A., Walker, A. S., Dorrucci, M., Sabin, C., Phillips, A., Porter, K., & CASCADE Collaboration. (2008). Changes in the incidence and predictors of human immunodeficiency virus-associated dementia in the era of highly active antiretroviral therapy. *Annals of Neurology, 63*(2), 213-221. https://doi.org/10.1002/ana.21225.

Boulware, D. R., Meya, D. B., Muzoora, C., Rolfes, M. A., Huppler Hullsiek, K., Musubire, A., Taseera, K., Nabeta, H. W., Schutz, C., Williams, D. A., Rajasingham, R., Rhein, J., Thienemann, F., Lo, M. W., Nielsen, K., Bergemann, T. L., Kambugu, A., Manabe, Y. C., Janoff, E. N., Bohjanen, P. R., & Meintjes, G.; COAT Trial Team. (2014). Timing of antiretroviral therapy after diagnosis of cryptococcal meningitis. *New England Journal of Medicine, 370*(26), 2487-2498. https://doi.org/10.1056/NEJMoa1312884.

Boulware, D. R., Rolfes, M. A., Rajasingham, R., von Hohenberg, M., Qin, Z., Taseera, K., Schutz, C., Kwizera, R., Butler, E. K., Meintjes, G., Muzoora, C., Bischof, J. C., & Meya, D. B. (2014). Multisite validation of cryptococcal antigen lateral flow assay and quantification by laser thermal contrast. *Emerging Infectious Diseases, 20*(1), 45-53. https://doi.org/10.3201/eid2001.130906.

Chappell, E. T., Guthrie, B. L., & Orenstein, J. (1992). The role of stereotactic biopsy in the management of HIV-related focal brain lesions. *Neurosurgery, 30*(6), 825-829. https://doi.org/10.1227/00006123-199206000-00001.

Cherner, M., Ellis, R. J., Lazzaretto, D., Young, C., Mindt, M. R., Atkinson, J. H., Grant, I., Heaton, R. K.; HIV Neurobehavioral Research Center Group. (2004). Effects of HIV-1 infection and aging on neurobehavioral functioning: preliminary findings. *AIDS, 18*, 27-34. https://doi.org/10.1097/00002030-200418001-00005.

Clifford, D. B., Arribas, J. R., Storch, G. A., Tourtellote, W., & Wippold, F. J. (1996). Magnetic resonance brain imaging lacks sensitivity for AIDS-associated cytomegalovirus encephalitis. *Journal of Neurovirology, 2*(6), 397-403. https://doi.org/10.3109/13550289609146905.

Cooley, S. A., Jeremy, F., Boerwinkle, A., Kilgore, C., & Beau, M. (2021). Effects of anticholinergic medication use on brain integrity in persons living with HIV and persons without HIV. *AIDS (London, England), 35*(3), 381. https://doi.org/10.1097/QAD.0000000000002768.

Coté, T. R., Biggar, R. J., Rosenberg, P. S., Devesa, S. S., Percy, C., Yellin, F. J., Lemp, G., Hardy, C., Geodert, J. J., Blattner, W. A. (1997). Non-Hodgkin's lymphoma among people with AIDS: incidence, presentation and public health burden.

International Journal of Cancer, 73(5), 645-650. https://doi.org/10.1002/(SICI)1097-0215(19971127)73:5<645::AID-IJC6>3.0.CO;2-X.

Cox, G. M., Perfect, J. R. (1997). *Cryptococcus neoformans var neoformans* and *gattii* and *Trichosporon* species. In: Edward LA (Ed), *Topley and Wilson's Microbiology and Microbial Infections* (9th Ed). London: Arnold Press.

d'Arminio Monforte, A., Cinque, P., Mocroft, A., Goebel, F. D., Antunes, F., Katlama, C., Justesen, U. S., Vella, S., Kirk, O., Lundgren, J.; EuroSIDA Study Group. (2004). Changing incidence of central nervous system diseases in the EuroSIDA cohort. *Annals of Neurology: Official Journal of the American Neurological Association and the Child Neurology Society, 55*(3), 320-328. https://doi.org/10.1002/ana.10827.

Dal Pan, G. J., McArthur, J. H., Aylward, E., Selnes, O. A., Nance-Sproson, T. E., Kumar, A. J., Mellits, E. D., McArthur, J. C. (1992). Patterns of cerebral atrophy in HIV-1-infected individuals: Results of a quantitative MRI analysis. *Neurology, 42*(11), 2125-2125. https://doi.org/10.1212/WNL.42.11.2125.

Darras-Joly, C., Chevret, S., Wolff, M., Matheron, S., Longuet, P., Casalino, E., Joly, V., Chochillon, C., Bédos, J. P. (1996). Cryptococcus neoformans infection in France: epidemiologic features of and early prognostic parameters for 76 patients who were infected with human immunodeficiency virus. *Clinical Infectious Diseases, 23*(2), 369-376. https://doi.org/10.1093/clinids/23.2.369.

Demir, S., Karakaş, E., Karakaş, Ö., & Koruk, S. T. (2013). Tüberküloz menenjit tanısında Manyetik Rezonans Görüntülemenin rolü [Role of Magnetic Resonance Imaging in the diagnosis of tuberculosis meningitis]. *Journal of Harran University Medical Faculty, 10*(2), 95-98.

Dunfee, R. L., Thomas, E. R., Gorry, P. R., Wang, J., Taylor, J., Kunstman, K., Wolinsky, S. M., & Gabuzda, D. (2006). The HIV Env variant N283 enhances macrophage tropism and is associated with brain infection and dementia. *Proceedings of the National Academy of Sciences, 103*(41), 15160-15165. https://doi.org/10.1073/pnas.0605513103.

Edén, A., Fuchs, D., Hagberg, L., Nilsson, S., Spudich, S., Svennerholm, B., Price, R. W., & Gisslén, M. (2010). HIV-1 viral escape in cerebrospinal fluid of subjects on suppressive antiretroviral treatment. *Journal of Infectious Diseases, 202*(12), 1819-1825. https://doi.org/10.1086/657342.

Edén, A., Price, R. W., Spudich, S., Fuchs, D., Hagberg, L., & Gisslén, M. (2007). Immune activation of the central nervous system is still present after > 4 years of effective highly active antiretroviral therapy. *Journal of Infectious Diseases, 196*(12), 1779-1783. https://doi.org/10.1086/523648.

Flood, J., Drew, W. L., Miner, R., Jekic-McMullen, D., Shen, L. P., Kolberg, J., Garvey, J., Follansbee, S., & Poscher, M. (1997). Diagnosis of cytomegalovirus (CMV) polyradiculopathy and documentation of in vivo anti-CMV activity in cerebrospinal fluid by using branched DNA signal amplification and antigen assays. *Journal of Infectious Diseases, 176*(2), 348-352. https://doi.org/10.1086/514051.

Gallant, J. E., Moore, R. D., Richman, D. D., Keruly, J., & Chaisson, R. E. (1992). the Zidovudine Epidemiology Study Group: Incidence and natural history of cytomegalovirus disease in patients with advanced human immunodeficiency virus disease treated with zidovudine. *J Infect Dis, 166*, 1223-1227. https://doi.org/10.1093/infdis/166.6.1223.

Garlipp, C. R., Rossi, C. L., & Bottini, P. V. (1997). Cerebrospinal fluid profiles in acquired immunodeficiency syndrome with and without neurocryptococcosis. *Revista do Instituto de Medicina Tropical de São Paulo, 39*, 323-326. https://doi.org/10.1590/S0036-46651997000600003.

Ghanem, K. G. (2010). Neurosyphilis: a historical perspective and review. *CNS Neuroscience & Therapeutics, 16*(5), e157-e168. https://doi.org/10.1111/j.1755-5949.2010.00183.x.

Gonzalez, E., Rovin, B. H., Sen, L., Cooke, G., Dhanda, R., Mummidi, S., Kulkarni, H., Bamshad, M. J., Telles, V., Anderson, S. A., Walter, E. A., Stephan, K. T., Deucher, M., Mangano, A., Bologna, R., Ahuja, S. S., Dolan, M. J., & Ahuja, S. K. (2002). HIV-1 infection and AIDS dementia are influenced by a mutant MCP-1 allele linked to increased monocyte infiltration of tissues and MCP-1 levels. *Proceedings of the National Academy of Sciences, 99*(21), 13795-13800. https://doi.org/10.1073/pnas.202357499.

Grill, M. F., & Price, R. W. (2014). Central nervous system HIV-1 infection. *Handbook of Clinical Neurology, 123*, 487-505. https://doi.org/10.1016/B978-0-444-53488-0.00023-7.

Gürses, C., Bilgiç, B., Topçular, B., Tuncer, O. G., Akman-Demir, G., Hanağası, H., Baslo, B., Gürvit, H., Coban, O., Emre, M., & Idrisoğlu, H. A. (2007). Clinical and magnetic resonance imaging findings of HIV-negative patients with neurosyphilis. *Journal of Neurology, 254*, 368-374. https://doi.org/10.1007/s00415-006-0380-z.

Heaton, R. K., Ellis, R. J., Tang, B., Marra, C. M., Rubin, L. H., Clifford, D. B., McCutchan, J. A., Gelman, B. B., Morgello, S., Franklin, D. R., & Letendre, S. L. (2023). Twelve-year neurocognitive decline in HIV is associated with comorbidities, not age: a CHARTER study. *Brain, 146*(3), 1121-1131. https://doi.org/10.1093/brain/awac465.

Johnson, B. A., Fram, E. K., Johnson, P. C., & Jacobowitz, R. (1997). The variable MR appearance of primary lymphoma of the central nervous system: comparison with histopathologic features. *American Journal of Neuroradiology, 18*(3), 563-572.

Jones, J. L., & Roberts, J. M. (2012). Toxoplasmosis hospitalizations in the United States, 2008, and trends, 1993-2008. *Clinical Infectious Diseases, 54*(7), e58-e61. https://doi.org/10.1093/cid/cir990.

Karl-Erık, Å., Ellıott, L. M., & Edward, P. R. (1958). Progressive multifocal leuko-encephalopathy. *Brain*, *81*(1), 93-111.10.1093/brain/81.1.93.

Lanoy, E., Guiguet, M., Bentata, M., Rouveix, E., Dhiver, C., Poizot-Martin, I., Costagliola, D., & Gasnault, J. (2011). Survival after neuroAIDS: association with antiretroviral CNS Penetration-Effectiveness score. *Neurology, 76*(7), 644-651. https://doi.org/10.1212/WNL.0b013e31820c3089.

Laskus, T., Radkowski, M., Bednarska, A., Wilkinson, J., Adair, D., Nowicki, M., Nikolopoulou, G. B., Vargas, H., & Rakela, J. (2002). Detection and analysis of hepatitis C virus sequences in cerebrospinal fluid. *Journal of virology, 76*(19), 10064-10068. https://doi.org/10.1128/JVI.76.19.10064-10068.2002.

Lee, S. C., Dickson, D. W., & Casadevall, A. (1996). Pathology of cryptococcal meningoencephalitis: analysis of 27 patients with pathogenetic implications. *Human pathology, 27*(8), 839-847. https://doi.org/10.1016/S0046-8177(96)90459-1.

Lescure, F. X., Moulignier, A., Savatovsky, J., Amiel, C., Carcelain, G., Molina, J. M., Gallien, S., Pacanovski, J., Pialoux, G., Adle-Biassette, H., & Gray, F. (2013). CD8 encephalitis in HIV-infected patients receiving cART: a treatable entity. *Clinical infectious diseases, 57*(1), 101-108. https://doi.org/10.1093/cid/cit175.

Liu, Y. T., Yang, T. C., Jung, S. M., & Lee, C. C. (2018). Probable pathogenesis, diagnosis, and management of untreated arteriovenous malformation with cyst formation: case report and literature review. *Acta Neurologica Belgica, 118*, 603-605. https://doi.org/10.1007/s13760-018-1011-z.

McCutchan, J. A., Marquie-Beck, J. A., Fitzsimons, C. A., Letendre, S. L., Ellis, R. J., Heaton, R. K., Wolfson, T., Rosario, D., Alexander, T. J., Marra, C., Ances, B. M., & Grant, I. (2012). Role of obesity, metabolic variables, and diabetes in HIV-associated neurocognitive disorder. *Neurology, 78*(7), 485-492. https://doi.org/10.1212/WNL.0b013e3182478d64.

McCutchan, J. A., Wu, J. W., Robertson, K., Koletar, S. L., Ellis, R. J., Cohn, S., Levine, A. J., Minagar, A., Novembre, F. J., Somboonwit, C., Nath, A., & Williams, P. L. (2007). HIV suppression by HAART preserves cognitive function in advanced, immune-reconstituted AIDS patients. *Aids, 21*(9), 1109-1117. https://doi.org/10.1097/QAD.0b013e3280ef6acd.

Mirza, S. A., Phelan, M., Rimland, D., Graviss, E., Hamill, R., Brandt, M. E., Gardner, T., Sattah, M., de Leon, G. P., Baughman, W., & Hajjeh, R. A. (2003). The changing epidemiology of cryptococcosis: an update from population-based active surveillance in 2 large metropolitan areas, 1992-2000. *Clinical infectious diseases, 36*(6), 789-794. https://doi.org/10.1086/368091.

Montoya, J. G., & Remington, J. S. (2000). *Toxoplasma gondii*. In: Mandell, G. L., Bennett, J. E., Dolin, R. (Eds), *Principles and Practice of Infectious Diseases (5th Edition, p.2858)*. Churchill Livingstone, Philadelphia.

Morgello, S., Cho, E. S., Nielsen, S., Devinsky, O., & Petito, C. K. (1987). Cytomegalovirus encephalitis in patients with acquired immunodeficiency syndrome: an autopsy study of 30 cases and a review of the literature. *Human pathology, 18*(3), 289-297. https://doi.org/10.1016/S0046-8177(87)80012-6.

Moulignier, A., Lamirel, C., Picard, H., Lebrette, M. G., Amiel, C., Hamidi, M., Polivka, M., Mikol, J., Cochereau, I., & Pialoux, G. (2017). Long-term AIDS-related PCNSL outcomes with HD-MTX and combined antiretroviral therapy. *Neurology, 89*(8), 796-804. https://doi.org/10.1212/WNL.0000000000004265.

Moulignier, A., & Costagliola, D. (2020). Metabolic syndrome and cardiovascular disease impacts on the pathophysiology and phenotype of HIV-associated neurocognitive disorders. In *Neurocognitive Complications of HIV-Infection: Neuropathogenesis to Implications for Clinical Practice* (pp. 367-399). Springer. https://doi.org/10.1007/7854_2019_123.

Murakawa, G. J., Kerschmann, R., & Berger, T. (1996). Cutaneous Cryptococcus infection and AIDS: report of 12 cases and review of the literature. *Archives of dermatology, 132*(5), 545-548. https://doi.org/10.1001/archderm.1996.03890290079010.

National Institutes of Health (2023). *Guidelines for the Prevention and Treatment of Opportunistic Infections in Adults and Adolescents with HIV: Toxoplasma gondii Encephalitis.* Retrieved from https://clinicalinfo.hiv.gov/en/guidelines/adult-and-adolescent-opportunistic-infection/toxoplasma-gondii-encephalitis (Accessed on April 20, 2023).

Peluso, M. J., Ferretti, F., Peterson, J., Lee, E., Fuchs, D., Boschini, A., Gisslén, M., Angoff, N., Price, R. W., Cinque, P., & Spudich, S. (2012). Cerebrospinal fluid HIV escape associated with progressive neurologic dysfunction in patients on antiretroviral therapy with well controlled plasma viral load. *Aids, 26*(14), 1765-1774. https://doi.org/10.1097/QAD.0b013e328355e6b2.

Porter, S. B., & Sande, M. A. (1992). Toxoplasmosis of the central nervous system in the acquired immunodeficiency syndrome. *New England Journal of Medicine, 327*(23), 1643-1648. https://doi.org/10.1056/NEJM199212033272306.

Raez, L. E., Patel, P., Feun, L., Restrepo, A., Raub Jr, W. A., & Cassileth, P. A. (1998). Natural history and prognostic factors for survival in patients with acquired immune deficiency syndrome (AIDS)-related primary central nervous system lymphoma (PCNSL). *Critical reviews in oncogenesis, 9*(3-4), 199-208.

Rajasingham, R., Smith, R. M., Park, B. J., Jarvis, J. N., Govender, N. P., Chiller, T. M., Denning, D. W., Loyse, A., Boulware, D. R. (2017). Global burden of disease of HIV-associated cryptococcal meningitis: an updated analysis. *The Lancet infectious diseases, 17*(8), 873-881. https://doi.org/10.1016/S1473-3099(17)30243-8.

Renold, C., Sugar, A., Chave, J. P., Perrin, L., Delavelle, J., Pizzolato, G., Burkhard, P., Gabriel, V., Hirschel, B. (1992). Toxoplasma encephalitis in patients with the acquired immunodeficiency syndrome. *Medicine, 71*(4), 224-239. https://doi.org/10.1097/00005792-199207000-00005.

Roc, A. C., Ances, B. M., Chawla, S., Korczykowski, M., Wolf, R. L., Kolson, D, Detre JA, Poptani, H. (2007). Detection of human immunodeficiency virus-induced inflammation and oxidative stress in lenticular nuclei with magnetic resonance spectroscopy despite antiretroviral therapy. *Archives of neurology, 64*(9), 1249-1257. https://doi.org/10.1001/archneur.64.9.noc60125.

Rubin, L. H., Radtke, K. K., Eum, S., Tamraz, B., Kumanan, K. N., Springer, G., Maki, P. M., Anastos, K., Merenstein, D., Karim, R., Weber, K. M., Gustafson, D., Greenblatt, R. M., Bishop, J. R. (2018). Cognitive burden of common non-antiretroviral medications in HIV-infected women. *Journal of acquired immune deficiency syndromes (1999), 79*(1), 83. https://doi.org/10.1097/QAI.0000000000001755.

Sacktor, N. (2002). The epidemiology of human immunodeficiency virus-associated neurological disease in the era of highly active antiretroviral therapy. *Journal of neurovirology, 8*(Suppl 2), *115-21.* https://doi.org/10.1080/13550280290101094.

Said, G., Lacroix, C., Chemouilli, P., Goulon-Goeau, C., Roullet, E., Penaud, D., de Broucker, T., Meduri, G., Vincent, D., Torchet, M., Leport, C., Vildé, J. L. (1991). Cytomegalovirus neuropathy in acquired immunodeficiency syndrome: a clinical and pathological study. *Annals of Neurology: Official Journal of the American Neurological Association and the Child Neurology Society, 29*(2), 139-146. https://doi.org/10.1002/ana.410290205.

San-Andrés, F. J., Rubio, R., Castilla, J., Pulido, F., Palao, G., de Pedro, I., Costa, J. R., del Palacio, A. (2003). Incidence of acquired immunodeficiency syndrome-associated opportunistic diseases and the effect of treatment on a cohort of 1115 patients infected with human immunodeficiency virus, 1989-1997. *Clinical infectious diseases, 36*(9), 1177-1185. https://doi.org/10.1086/374358.

Schouten, J., Cinque, P., Gisslen, M., Reiss, P., & Portegies, P. (2011). HIV-1 infection and cognitive impairment in the cART era: a review. *Aids, 25*(5), 561-575. https://doi.org/10.1097/QAD.0b013e3283437f9a.

Schwarcz, L., Chen, M. J., Vittinghoff, E., Hsu, L., & Schwarcz, S. (2013). Declining incidence of AIDS-defining opportunistic illnesses: results from 16 years of population-based AIDS surveillance. *Aids, 27*(4), 597-605. https://doi.org/10.1097/QAD.0b013e32835b0fa2.

Shapshak, P., Kangueane, P., Fujimura, R. K., Commins, D., Chiappelli, F., Singer, E., Levine, A. J., Minagar, A., Novembre, F. J., Somboonwit, C., Nath, A., & Sinnott, J. T. (2011). Editorial neuroAIDS review. *AIDS (London, England), 25*(2), 123. https://doi.org/10.1097/QAD.0b013e328340fd42.

Price, R. W. (1996). Neurological complications of HIV infection. *The Lancet, 348*(9025), 445-452. https://doi.org/10.1016/S0140-6736(95)11035-6.

Sünbül, M. (2003). Tüberküloz Menenjit [Tuberculosıs Menıngıtıs]. *21st Century Tuberculosis Symposium and II. Tuberculosis Laboratory Diagnostic Methods Course*, Samsun. Retrieved from https://www.klimik.org.tr/wp-content/uploads/2012/02/982011124450-Mustafa_Sunbul.pdf.

Thurnher, M. M., Thurnher, S. A., & Schindler, E. (1997). CNS involvement in AIDS: spectrum of CT and MR findings. *European radiology, 7*, 1091-1097. https://doi.org/10.1007/s003300050260.

Valcour, V., Yee, P., Williams, A. E., Shiramizu, B., Watters, M., Selnes, O., Paul, R., Shikuma, C., & Sacktor, N. (2006). Lowest ever CD4 lymphocyte count (CD4 nadir) as a predictor of current cognitive and neurological status in human immunodeficiency virus type 1 infection-The Hawaii Aging with HIV Cohort. *Journal of neurovirology, 12*, 387-391. https://doi.org/10.1080/13550280600915339.

Wohrl, S., & Geusau, A. (2006). Neurosyphilis is unlikely in patients with late latent syphilis and a negative blood VDRL test. *Acta Dermatovenereologica-Stockholm, 86*(4), 335. https://doi.org/10.2340/00015555-0092.

Chapter 15

Fungal CNS Infections

Sema Tekin Şahin*, MD

Department of Infectious Diseases and Clinical Microbiology,
Alanya Training and Research Hospital, Antalya, Turkiye

Abstract

With the emergence of the human immunodeficiency virus epidemic and the increasing use of immunosuppressive drugs, the incidence of deep mycoses has increased, as has the range of fungi causing potentially lethal diseases. These developments have come together to make it critical for physicians to increase their knowledge and understanding of medically important fungi (Bennett et al., 2015, p. 2874). Infections of the central nervous system (CNS) caused by fungi can broadly be divided into those that affect immunocompetent hosts (Cryptococcus, Coccidioides, Histoplasma, Blastomyces, and Sporothrix species) and those that affect immunocompromised hosts (Candida, Aspergillus, Zygomycetes, and Trichosporon species) as opportunistic infections (Woods et al., 2007). Despite being uncommon, fungus infections of the CNS have increased in frequency during the last few decades (Raman Sharma, 2010). This is primarily due to the increased use of immunosuppressive therapies, improvements made in stem cell and organ transplantation, and the spread of HIV/AIDS (Nathan et al., 2021). In immunocompromised hosts, fungal infections cause significant morbidity, and involvement of the CNS could be fatal. In general, compared to viral, bacterial, or parasitic CNS disorders, symptomatic fungal infection has a higher risk of morbidity and mortality. Thus, early detection and appropriate medical and surgical management strategies are critical in improving the overall prognosis of CNS mycosis (Raman Sharma, 2010).

* Corresponding Author's Email: sematekinsahin@gmail.com.

In: Central Nervous System Infections
Editor: Mustafa Usanmaz
ISBN: 979-8-89113-660-1

Keywords: fungal infections, antifungal treatment, central nervous system infections

Introduction

At present, over 100,000 different fungus species have been identified, however, only a small proportion of these have been shown to be pathogenic, and around 10-15% of them cause neurological disease (Nathan et al., 2021). Pathogenic fungal species can infect both immunocompromised and immunocompetent patients. In immunocompetent individuals, disease-causing species show a limited geographic distribution, while opportunistic pathogenic fungal species are found all over the world. Species with limited geographic distribution occur mostly in North America; these are Blastomycetes, Coccidioides, Paracoccidioides, Histoplasma, and Sporothrix. Opportunistic pathogenic fungi species are Aspergillus, Candida, Cryptococcus, and Rhizopus.

The two primary routes by which mycoses are transmitted through direct contact with and inhaling fungus spores into the paranasal sinuses. Fungi spread and enter the CNS through the bloodstream when fungal clearance fails at the location of the initial infection (Panackal and Williamson, 2015, p.1662-1678). Candida albicans enter the intestinal and mucosal microbiome during birth or later in life through contact with colonized people.

Minor trauma to saprophytic fungus on plants or soil can result in chromoblastomycosis, sporotrichosis, or mycetoma. Ingestion has not been shown to be a pathway for pathogenic fungi. Water contact is suspected of transmitting rhinosporidiosis.

Coccidioidomycosis, Histoplasmosis, cryptococcosis, and blastomycosis agents grow in the environment, are inhaled, and cause infection in the lungs. The spatial constraint of these mycoses is due to a constrained reservoir in nature (Bennett et al., 2015, p.2878).

Fungi spread and enter the CNS through the bloodstream when fungal clearance fails at the location of the initial infection (Panackal and Williamson, 2015, p.1662-1678).

Patients who are immunocompromised, elderly, or undergoing neurological surgery are highly susceptible to fungal central nervous system infections, and failure to seek prompt diagnosis and treatment can be fatal for such patients. The fungi that cause CNS infections the most often are reviewed in Table 1.

Table 1. Fungal infections of the central nervous system: epidemiology and clinical manifestations (Bloch and Bailin, 2019, p. 278)

Class	Organism	Emerging Species	Geographic Distribution	Major Risk Factors	Clinical Presentation
Molds	Aspergillus spp.		World-wide	Hematologic malignancies, solid organ transplant, steroids, neurosurgery	Brain abscess, rhinocerebral infection, meningitis, CNS vasculitis
	Mucorales		World-wide	Diabetes mellitus, iron overload, hematologic malignancies, steroids	Rhinocerebral infection, brain abscess
Yeasts	Candida spp	C.auris	World-wide	Preterm birth, neurosurgery, steroids, injection drug use, chronic liver disease	Meningitis
	Cryptococcal spp	C.gattii	C. neoformans world-wide C. gattii-Asia, British Columbia, Pacific NW, SE US	AIDS, steroids, solid organ transplant, liver disease	Meningitis
			C. gattii-Asia, British Columbia, Pacific NW, SE US	C gattii infections are more frequent in immunocompetent host	
Dimorphic Fungi	Blastomyces	B. gilchristii	US, East of the Mississippi River	TNF-alpha inhibitors, steroids, HIV/AIDS. Approximately 50% immunocompetent	Meningitis, brain abscess
	Coccidioides	C. posadasii	Western US	HIV/AIDS, steroids, Filipino or African descent. Approximately 3/4 of cases without predisposing cause	Meningitis, CNS vasculitis
	Histoplasma		US East of the Mississippi River	HIV/AIDS, steroids, transplant, TNF-alpha inhibitors. Approximately 30% of cases of immunocompetent	Meningitis

Cryptococcus

Before 1955, there had been only 300 cryptococcosis cases described in the literature. The encapsulated, hetero-basidiomycetous fungi Cryptococcus neoformans and Cryptococcus gattii have evolved from being uncommon human pathogens to common, global opportunistic pathogens, as immunocompromised human populations have increased dramatically over the past 20 years (Park et al., 2019).

While C. gattii is mostly found in tropical and subtropical trees and eucalyptus in Papua New Guinea, Australia, Southern California, parts of Africa, the Pacific Northwest region of the USA, Mexico and British Columbia, C. neoformans has a worldwide distribution linked to the presence of pigeon excrement (Kohler et al., 2014; Harris et al., 2012).

A well-defined underlying immunocompromised state is present in the great majority of patients with symptomatic disseminated cryptococcosis. AIDS, extended corticosteroid therapy, organ transplantation, advanced cancer, diabetes, and sarcoidosis are among the most prevalent underlying diseases in the world (Bennett et al., 2015, p.2937). Although most of the patients are immunosuppressed, around 20% of people with cryptococcosis who are not HIV-positive are thought to be free of any underlying conditions or risk factors.

The two distinctive features of C. gattii and C. neoformans are the polysaccharide capsule and the production of melanin. The effects of capsular polysaccharide on host immunity can be significant at several pathophysiological levels. It has been demonstrated to have the following impacts on the host: (1) it functions as an anti-phagocytosis barrier (2) it decreases complement (3) it disrupts the secretion of cytokines (4) it causes antibody nonresponsiveness (5) it interferes with antigen presentation (6) it causes brain edema (7) it enables a highly negative charge to surrounding yeast cells (8) it leads to selectin and tumor necrosis factor receptor loss (9) it improves HIV replication, and (10) it extrudes itself into the intracellular environment with the potential for local toxicity on cellular organelles (Casadevall and Perfect, 1998). Melanin production as another virulence factor also has protective mechanisms. These are (1) support or integrity of the cell wall; (2) durability against temperature changes and antifungal medications; (3) disruption of the T-cell response; (4) elimination of antibody-mediated phagocytosis; and (5) change in the charge of the cell wall (Bennett et al., 2015, p.2939).

Lungs are the site of the first infection; however, the infection subsequently frequently spreads to other organs, primarily through lymphatic and hematogenous routes, potentially involving internal organs and the central nervous system (Murthy and Sundaram, 2014; Harris et al., 2012).

The two most common sites of cryptococcal infections are the lungs and the central nervous system. The majority of individuals with CNS cryptococcosis initially display symptoms of subacute meningitis, such as cranial nerve palsies, lethargy, headache, coma, fever, or memory loss over a period of weeks. Patients may arrive with symptoms that are not usual, such as acute (lasting many days) symptoms of intermittent headaches, severe headaches, or possibly no symptoms at all but with a changed mental state (Perfect, 1989). Intracranial mass lesions, also known as cryptococcomas, are an extremely rare symptom of cerebral cryptococcosis. MRI-based amplification of mass lesions in the form of rings, with or without cystic alterations, may be an indicator of cryptococcoma. Lesions are more seldom encountered in the intraspinal region and pons, with the basal ganglia, cerebellum, or parietal lobe being the most frequent sites (Figure 1) (Li et al., 2009; Velmakanni et al., 2014).

The diagnosis of CNS cryptococcal infections is based on microscopic examination, culture, antigen detection, and radiology. A quick and reliable way to diagnose cryptococcal meningitis is still to mix India ink and cerebrospinal fluid to look for the 5- to 10-micron-diameter encapsulated yeasts (Bennett et al., 2015, p. 2944). India ink staining is positive in 80% of patients with concurrent AIDS but is less prevalent in immunocompetent people (50%) (Perfect et al., 1983). The gold standard for diagnosing cryptococcal CNS infection is to isolate the yeast with culture. On the majority of bacterial and fungal mediums, C. neoformans can grow. Automated and lysis centrifugation techniques work well for detecting cryptococcemia. The majority of C. neoformans strains from untreated individuals can be found in culture three to seven days after the material is obtained and put into or on culture medium. There may be over one million colony-forming organisms of yeast per milliliter of cerebrospinal fluid (CSF) in some severe CNS infections (Bicanic et al., 2009) (Figure 2).

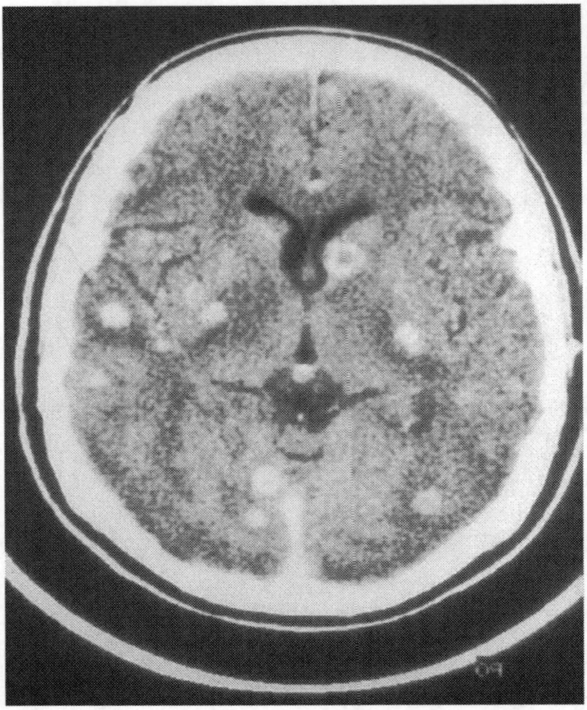

Figure 1. CT imaging of a patient with numerous cryptococcomas who was previously healthy (Li et al., 2009; Velmakanni et al., 2014).

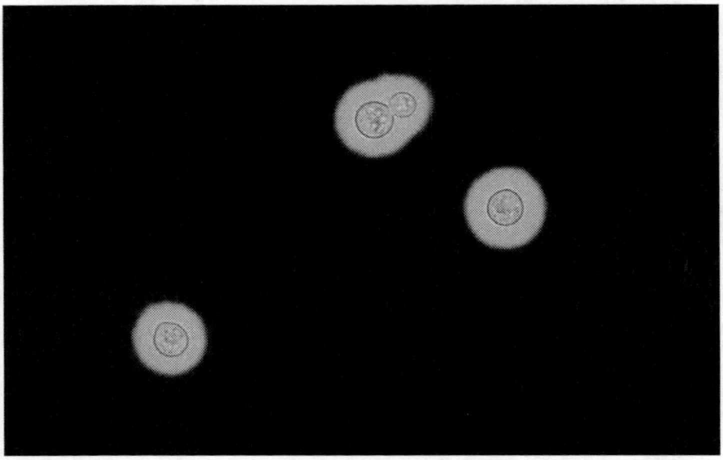

Figure 2. India ink preparations obtained from the CSF of a patient with meningitis (notice the yeasts that are encapsulated (Bennett et al., 2015, p.2944).

Cryptococcal polysaccharide antigen detection techniques in CSF and serum are very effective in detecting invasive disease (Goodman et al., 1971). Both the latex agglutination (LA) and enzyme-linked immunosorbent test (ELISA) assays have sensitivity and specificity greater than 90%. The sensitivity and specificity of latex agglutination (LA) and enzyme-linked immunosorbent assay (ELISA) assays are both better than 90% (Kauffman et al., 1981). Even three weeks before meningitis symptoms appear, the serum can be used to perform a lateral assay test. Since 2018, WHO recommendations have advised that all adults and children living with HIV with a CD4 cell count of 100 cells/mm3 undergo a cryptococcal antigen screening prior to starting or restarting ART; cryptococcal antigen testing may also be taken into consideration for adults and children with HIV who have a CD4 cell count of less than 200 cells/mm3.

In radiological imaging, non-contrast tomography can be found to be normal in cryptococcal infection. MR imaging, on the other hand, can detect more findings. The MRI of cryptococcal meningoencephalitis reveals generalized meningeal enhancement and ventriculitis. Due to the cryptococcal invasion of the Virchow-Robin spaces, the characteristic 'soap bubble lesions' are punctate, cystic lesions most commonly found in the basal ganglia. These lesions can even become ring-enhancing in patients with immune reconstitution syndrome. Moreover, lacunar strokes in the basal ganglia, a kind of ischemic stroke, are seen more frequently with cryptococcal meningitis (Vela-Duarte et al., 2019).

In the treatment of CNS cryptococcal infections, induction, maintenance, and consolidation treatment is required. The cornerstone of therapy for cryptococcal meningitis remains amphotericin B. For Amphotericin B deoxycholate, an induction dose of 0,7mg/kg/day is recommended. Treatment outcomes with amphotericin B lipid complex and liposomal amphotericin B at 3 to 6 mg/kg/day were comparable to those with amphotericin B deoxycholate, but with less toxicity (Leenders et al., 1997). Flucytosine should be used in conjunction with amphotericin B, not alone, due to the risk of drug resistance. Flucytosine is administered at a dosage of 100 mg/kg/day to individuals with normal renal function. To reduce the development of bone marrow depression, complete blood counts should be closely monitored (Stamm et al., 1987).

Two weeks of induction treatment with combination therapy of amfotericin B ve flusitozin are adequate if clinical response and CSF sterilization have been accomplished. For the maintenance treatment, fluconazole at 800 mg per day should be used until the CSF cultures are verified to be sterile. Relapses were more common in individuals receiving 400 mg fluconazole than in those receiving 800 mg, according to a phase 2 study of treatment (Pappas et al., 2009). The overall duration of consolidation treatment is also determined by clinical response, HIV status, and CSF sterilization. After maintenance, consolidation treatment should be continued to prevent relapses. With the 200 mg/daily dose of fluconazole, the relapse rates decreased below 5% (Bozzette et al., 1991). The criteria for discontinuing medication are not clearly defined, but symptoms remission, at least two negative CSF cultures, and normal CSF glucose or a prolonged asymptomatic interval of 6 months to 1 year should be maintained (Bennett et al., 2015, p.2947). It should also be underlined that antiretroviral therapy should be started after at least 4 weeks of induction therapy in order to avoid causing immune reconstitution syndrome (IRIS) in newly diagnosed HIV/AIDS patients. Elevated intracranial pressure must be treated in addition to anti-fungal and anti-retroviral medication with repeated lumbar punctures, lumbar drains, or ventricular shunting (Eisenman et al., 2007).

There are key prognostic findings for cryptococcal meningitis. Increased intracranial pressure, the existence of underlying comorbid disease, an elevated fungal content in the CSF, and a low state of consciousness at the time of diagnosis are associated with a poor prognosis (Woods et al., 2007). Tragically, the immediate death rate of cryptococcal meningitis (at 6 months to a year) in industrialized countries still ranges from 10% to 25% (Chayakulkeeree and Perfect, 2006; Singh et al., 1997). While in underdeveloped nations with insufficient resources, the mortality rate at 6 months can be as high as 100% (Mwaba et al., 2001).

Coccidioides

The dimorphic fungus Coccidioides spp. (Coccidioides immitis and posadasii) can be found as mycelia or as unique particles called spherules (Sun et al., 1979). Within the genus, there are two species: C. posadasii, which is more abundant in Central and South America, Texas, and C. immitis, which is more frequent in California. The clinical manifestations of the two species are the same.

Coccidioides spp. grow as mycelia in standard microbiologic nutrient agar medium and are most likely found in topsoils. 1 week of maturation results in arthroconidia that can survive for a long time and are susceptible to separation from each other by physical disturbance or little air turbulence. Furthermore, the outcome is arthroconidia become airborne. Once it is inhaled, the arthroconidia land in terminal bronchioles, where they develop into spherules, burst, release endospores, and then develop into spherules once again. Although the spherules are normally restricted to the lungs, they can move to other end organs through lymphatics or lymph hematogenously (Woods et al., 2007).

Coccidioides spp. cause infections that extend beyond the lungs in approximately 0.5% of all infections in the population as a whole. Immunodeficiency conditions (e.g., HIV/AIDS, Hodgkin lymphoma) and immunosuppressive therapies dramatically increase the risk of dissemination. Most sites of dissemination are skin, joints, and bones (Bennett et al., 2015, p.2979).

The most severe type of disseminated infection is coccidioidal meningitis. If left untreated, it is most often fatal within two years after diagnosis (Einstein et al., 1961; Vincent et al., 1993).

Signs and symptoms include photophobia, meningismus, encephalopathy, back discomfort, and vision or hearing problems (Kirkland and Fierer, 2018). Suppurative and granulomatous inflammation causes basilar meningitis, which impairs the flow of CSF, resulting in hydrocephalus.

For the diagnosis of coccidioidomycosis direct examination, culture, serologic testing, and complement-fixing antibodies can be used.

Direct examination of the CSF can be used for CNS infections. In coccidioidal meningitis, CSF observations include leukocyte pleocytosis that ranges from 20 to 2000 cells/L, which is generally lymphocytic but can be polymorphonuclear (Jackson et al., 2019). Cytology stains, hematoxylin, and eosin stains, along with other specialised techniques, such as periodic acid-Schiff or silver staining, can also reveal spherules (Bennett et al., 2015, p.2980) (Figure 3).

Complement-fixing antibodies seen in cerebrospinal fluid are indicative of coccidioidal meningitis. Complement-fixing antibodies were detected in the CSF of 70 out of 92 individuals with coccidioidal meningitis in early trials. Nevertheless, advances in technology, such as overnight cold incubation, have improved the result to 251 of 265 patients with coccidioidal meningitis (95% sensitivity) (Kelly, 1980).

MRI brain imaging, which is more sensitive than CT scanning, is also used with diagnosis. Findings suggesting meningitis include the development of the Sylvian fissures, basal cisterns, pericallosal regions, or craniocervical junction. The hydrocephalus-related features include dilated lateral ventricles, rounded and enlarged frontal horns, or enlarged and rounded temporal horns

(Arsura et al., 2005). In between 30% and 40% of patients, edema or acute deep cerebral infarcts are presented associated with meningitis or hydrocephalus.

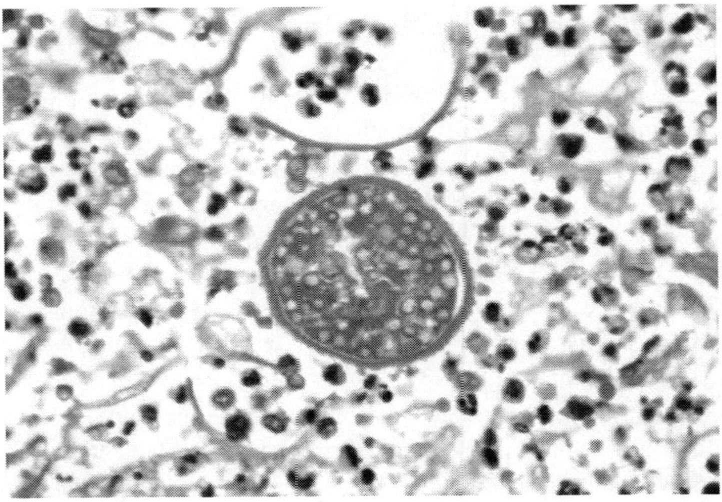

Figure 3. A spherule in a tissue, photographed under a microscope. Staining with hematoxylin and eosin (Courtesy Richard Sobonya, MD, University of Arizona) (Bennett et al., 2015, p.2975).

In contrast to other types of fungal meningitis such as cryptococcal meningitis, amphotericin B deoxycholate was shown to be ineffective in treating CNS infection when given intravenously (Stevens, 2001). Although intrathecal amphotericin B can be used in the treatment, there have been risks such as bleeding, arachnoiditis, and secondary bacterial infection (Goldstein et al., 2006). Furthermore, relapses are frequent when treatment is interrupted or discontinued, and the cure rate is only 30% (Kelly, 1980).

Fluconazole 800 mg daily is the current starting dose for treatment. Some healthcare professionals would reduce that amount to 400 mg/day after several months of therapy and improvement in clinical symptoms, while others would keep it at 800 mg daily. In any situation, with a recurrence rate of approximately 80%, if therapy is terminated, therapy would be continued indefinitely (Dewnsup, 1996).

In cases where fluconazole treatment is unsuccessful, several options are available. One of them is to increase the dose of fluconazole to 1200mg (Johnson et al., 2018), which will lead to an increase in side effects such as alopecia, hepatitis, and dry skin. The other option is to replace fluconazole therapy with posaconazole or voriconazole. According to recent data, Coccidioides is much less susceptible to fluconazole in vitro compared to other triazole antifungals (Thompson et al., 2017).

Histoplasmosis

Histoplasma capsulatum is a soil-based fungus that is currently identified throughout the world and is most commonly associated with valleys of rivers; the Ohio and Mississippi River Valleys are the most endemic (Bennett et al., 2015, p.2949).

It is typically found in soil and excavation or building of the soil is one of the most prevalent methods of releasing infectious particles that are inhaled and finally settle into the lungs. Because farming, spelunking, and demolition are all activities related to an elevated risk of exposure (Nathan et al., 2021).

The organism has two morphologies: mycelial and yeast phases. The mycelial form is present at room temperature, whereas the yeast form is present at 37°C or above. An examination of the mycelial phase under the microscope reveals two types of conidia. Macroconidia are large ovoid entities with diameters ranging from 8 to 15 μm. Microconidia are small smooth oval bodies that range in size from 2 to 5 μm. Since they are small enough to lodge in the terminal bronchioles and alveoli, microconidia are thought to be the infective phase (Figure 4) (Bennett et al., 2015, p.2951).

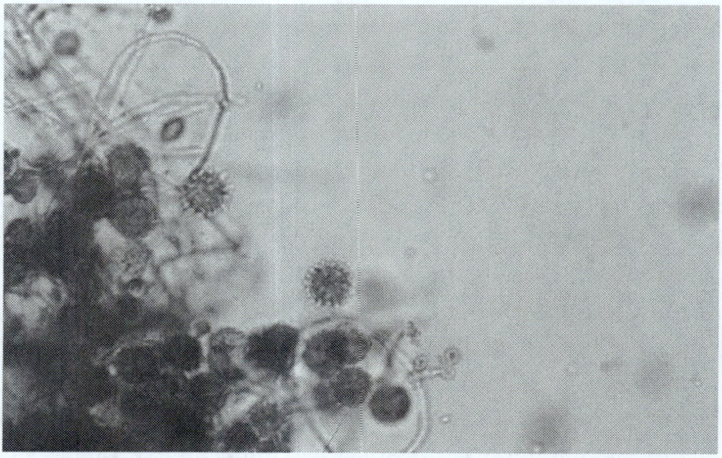

Figure 4. Histoplasma capsulatum mycelial phase. There are both macroconidia and microconidia present (Bennett et al., 2015, p.2951).

After the microconidia are inhaled, the conidia settle in the alveoli and transform from the saprophytic phase to the yeast phase. 90% of the primary infection in this way is asymptomatic or manifests as a flu-like disease and patients recover in about 14 days. However, in elderly patients, infants under two years of age, and immunocompromised patients, yeasts spread to distant organs via the lymphatic system and develop progressive disseminated disease symptoms.

Histoplasmosis can present in the CNS as a mass lesion and cerebritis, the most frequent of which is chronic meningitis. The most common symptoms were headache (60%) and disturbed mental state (42%). In 30% of the cases, focal neurological abnormalities were detected (Wheat et al., 2018).

In up to 60% of cases, the diagnosis of Histoplasma meningitis is frequently made later than one month and in rare cases only at autopsy (Wheat et al., 2018).

The primary cause of the delay is a lack of suspicion regarding a fungal origin. The CSF profile in CNS histoplasmosis is similar to that of other fungal meningitis. Typically, the CSF profile is characterized by monocytic pleocytosis, high protein, and low glucose. The definite diagnosis can be proven by isolation of Histoplasma capsulatum from tissues or bodily fluids. The standard medium used to isolate the fungus from sterile fluids is brain heart infusion agar. In most cultures, growth appears around three weeks, and in over 90% of cultures, the fungus appears around seven days (Bennett et al., 2015, p.2958). But in meningitis, in 25% to 65% of individuals, the organism is recovered from the CSF, and if a large amount of fluid (20 mL or more) is cultured and this percentage can be increased (Wheat et al., 2018).

Most of the time, the diagnosis can be made based on the finding of anti-Histoplasma antibodies or Histoplasma antigen in the CSF. Enzyme immunoassay (EIA), immunodiffusion (ID), and complement fixation (CF) are techniques for detecting antibodies. EIA was more sensitive (82%) than complement fixation (CF) (50%), ID (44%), or a combination of ID and CF (51%) for IgG and IgM anti-Histoplasma antibodies. With the EIA, the specificity was 93%, and, for immunodiffusion and complement fixation combined, it was 96% (Riddle and Wheat, 2019). According to a recent research study, the sensitivity for antigen detection in CSF was 78% and the specificity was 97%. (Bloch et al., 2017).

72% of the patients had abnormal brain imaging. The most frequently seen abnormality, present in 20% of patients, was focal mass lesions. Focal mass lesions, diffuse white matter alterations, low-density lesions in the cerebellum,

dizziness, fevers, lethargy, convulsions, and abnormal gait (Kourkoumpetis et al., 2012).

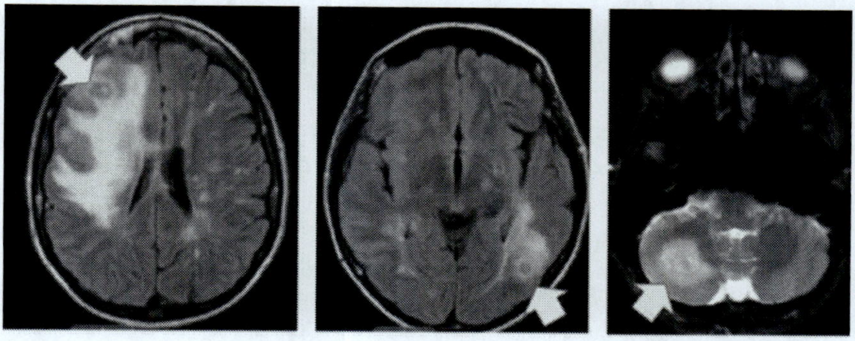

Figure 5. A 30-year-old female with proven cerebral aspergillosis was diagnosed 45 days after orthotopic liver transplantation. The T2 and FLAIR signal are hyperintense across the cerebral white matter in the left occipital lobe and right cerebellum, as well as deep gray nucleus structures with distinct ring-enhanced lesions and associated edema (arrows) (Miceli, 2019).

For a conclusive diagnosis of invasive aspergillosis, a tissue sample indicating infiltration of hyphae and a positive Aspergillus culture are required (De Pauw et al., 2008). Aspergillus successfully cultured on Sabourad's agar and exhibits distinctive conidiophores. CSF and blood cultures, nevertheless, are typically negative, even in cases of disseminated disease (Nadkarni and Goel, 2005).

Brain magnetic resonance imaging may reveal ring-enhancing lesions indicative of abscesses; however, critically immunocompromised individuals may have limited or even no contrast enhancement (Ruhnke et al., 2007). Additionally, ischemic infarcts with the potential for subsequent hemorrhagic transformation may be seen on MRI, and mycotic aneurysms may be detected with MR angiography (Nathan et al., 2021). Individuals with hematogenous spread may develop with solitary or numerous lesions at the gray-white junction, whereas individuals with aspergillosis of the CNS related to direct sinus invasion produce solitary lesions inside the temporal or frontal lobes (Starkey et al., 2014; Nadkarni and Goel, 2005).

Galactomannan (GM) is an ingredient in the polysaccharide cell-wall that is produced by the majority of Aspergillus spp. during hyphal growth. It can be identified using enzyme immunoassays (EIA) (Lamoth, 2016; Jenks and Hoenigl, 2020). Circulating GM could be positive days before the clinical symptoms of invasive aspergillosis, but as circulating GM in serum is intermittent, screening tests must be performed for a minimum of twice a week (Luckowitsch et al., 2021).

The presence of galactomannan antigen and 1,3--D-glucan in the CSF could be helpful in the diagnosis of aspergillosis in the CNS (Soeffker et al., 2013; Mikulska et al., 2013). Nevertheless, since 1,3--D-glucan and galactomannan antigen can be produced by fusarium species, their presence in the CSF is insufficient to support a diagnosis of aspergillosis in the CNS (Tortorano et al., 2012).

The three antifungal drug classes that can be utilized for managing aspergillosis are azoles, echinocandins, and polyenes. The right treatment for aspergillosis is dependent on the immunological condition of the host, the function of the kidneys and liver, previous treatments, and the possibility of a resistant infection (UpTodate, 2022).

Currently, the first-line treatment for most patients with invasive aspergillosis is voriconazole, which is a potent, broad-spectrum triazole (Walsh et al., 2008). Voriconazole has the broadest distribution in the CSF of any existing systemic antifungal, with CSF concentrations approaching 50% of plasma levels (Schwartz and Thiel, 2009). The regular IV loading of voriconazole is two doses of 6 mg/kg every 12 hours, followed by two doses of 4 mg/kg every 12 hours. Oral loading is 400 mg Q12 h 2 doses, then 200 mg PO q 12 h. The duration of antifungal therapy is not precisely determined and often lasts many months, depending on radiological and clinical response and continued immunosuppression (Miceli, 2019) (Table 2). In most cases, voriconazole is well tolerated. A temporary and transitory vision impairment is recorded by about 30% of individuals taking the medicine as the most prevalent side effect. It is dose-related and transient, with no pathogenic sequelae (Herbrecht et al., 2002). Therefore, voriconazole therapeutic drug monitoring has been advocated with the intention of limiting side effects that are shown to be more prevalent at concentrations over 6μg/mL and lower effectiveness at concentrations lower than 1μg/mL (Pascual et al., 2012; Trifilio et al., 2007).

Posaconazole and isavuconazole are recommended substitutes for people who cannot tolerate voriconazole or to prevent its negative effects. In randomized studies, both have been proven to have similar efficacy as voriconazole and to have greater tolerability (Maretens et al., 2021; Maertens et al., 2016).

Table 2. Antifungal medications and penetration into the central nervous system (Miceli, 2019)

Antifungal Agent	Molecular Mass	Protein Binding	CSF Concentration*	Comment
Voriconazole	349 Daltons	58%	~50%	Small, mildly lipophilic molecule
Posaconazole	708 Daltons	>98%	Very low to undetectable	The largest lipophilic molecule, inadequate information
Itraconazole	705 Daltons	99.8%	<10%	Lipophilic molecule
Isavuconazole	437 Daltons	>99%	Low	Soluble in water High concentration in eyes and brain
Amphotericin B and lipid formulations	924 Daltons	90%	Poor in adults; 40–90% in neonates Limited data with lipid formulations	Large compound with a hydrophilic polydroxyl chain and a lipophilic polyene hydrocarbon chain, poorly soluble in water
Echinocandins	1140-1292 Daltons	97-99%	Negligible	Brain tissue concentration can increase with increasing doses and sustained exposure

*plasma concentration as a percentage, information from both human and animal studies.

When voriconazole cannot be used, amphotericin B (AmB) deoxycholate and its lipid derivatives are acceptable alternatives for the primary and rescue treatment of Aspergillus infections (Patterson et al., 2016). Amphotericin B lipid formulations are less likely to produce nephrotoxicity than amphotericin B deoxycholate.

Echinocandins are effective against Aspergillus species, however, their biodistribution to the eye and uninfected CSF is poor. Therefore, echinocandins are not advised for use in treating CNS aspergillosis (Miceli, 2019).

In addition to antifungal therapy, since individuals with chronic and severe immune dysfunction and organ illness that limits the administration of antifungal treatment had the worst outcomes (Sipsas and Kontoyiannis, 2006), immunosuppressive medication should be reduced or terminated whenever possible in the immunocompromised host with CNS infection (Nadkarni and Goel, 2005).

Colony-stimulating factors are not yet advised for routine therapy in neutropenic individuals with invasive aspergillosis (Patterson et al., 2016;

Safdar, 2013). Each situation should be examined individually to weigh the advantages and hazards.

When it is possible, surgical removal of infected tissue should be performed, including paranasal sinuses, bone, and brain abscesses. The size and location of the lesion(s), the extent of resection needed, comorbidities, performance status, the patient's capacity to tolerate surgery, and the underlying diseases all affect the decision to perform surgery (Patterson et al., 2016).

Candida

Ascomycetes of the genus Candida are the most frequently identified opportunistic fungus in humans (Góralska et al., 2018). The frequency of almost all types of Candida infections has increased sharply after the 1940s with the widespread use of antibiotics. For the last few decades, Candida spp. has been the fourth most frequent pathogen detected in the blood of hospitalized patients in the United States (Pappas, 2011). The number of Candida infections has increased due to the increasing incidence of human immunodeficiency virus-1 infection, the use of treatment methods for enhanced life support and specific surgical operations such as organ transplantation and the implant of prosthetic devices (Bennett et al., 2015, p.2879).

C. albicans organisms have been found in soil, animals, hospitals, inanimate objects, and food. Non-albicans species can exist in both animal and non-animal settings (Bennett et al., 2015, p.2880). Candida spp. may be part of the normal microbiota of the oral cavity, gastrointestinal system, and urogenital tract in immunocompetent people. However, they may over-proliferate and cause invasive candidiasis when the normal defense systems of the organism are impaired (Góralska et al., 2018).

Over the past two decades, the incidence of invasive candidiasis has increased by 15 to 20 times (Pappas et al., 2018). Furthermore, in certain hospitals, candidaemia has been identified as the leading cause of healthcare-associated bloodstream infection (Magill et al., 2014; Pfaller and Diekema, 2007). The indicators of risk for invasive candidiasis are advanced care of premature neonates, organ transplantation, extended stay in the intensive care unit, exposure to wide-spectrum antibiotics and cancer chemotherapy, major abdominal surgery, implanted medical devices such as vascular catheters and prosthetic heart valves, and intravenous nutrition (Ben-Ami, 2018).

In Candida infections, CNS involvement is the most common in individuals with disseminated candidiasis or those who have neurological surgery (Góralska et al., 2018). Candida infects the meninges, as well as the parenchymal brain tissue (Liu et al., 2011). When it infects the parenchyma, Candida is indicated multiple cerebral abscesses with nodular enhancing lesions or ring enhancement (Góralska et al., 2018). The most frequent clinical manifestation of neurocandidiasis is meningoencephalitis. Candida is the 3rd most prevalent causal agent of fungal meningoencephalitis, causing approximately 8% of cases after Cryptococcus spp. and Coccidioides immitis (Forster et al., 2022). Candida meningitis begins with symptoms similar to bacterial meningitis, including headache, changed mental status, fever, and neck rigidity. Candida meningitis, on the other hand, usually has through a subacute beginning, contrary to bacterial meningitis, which often has a more abrupt start (Sánchez–Portocarrero et al., 2000). The clinical signs of diffuse microabscesses involving the central nervous system could vary (Bennett et al., 2015, p.2885). When present, genuine Candida abscesses tend to affect the parieto-occipital region and exhibit focal neurologic symptoms or seizures (Sánchez–Portocarrero et al., 2000).

In any individual presenting neurological symptoms and an existing invasive Candida infection, invasion of the central nervous system by Candida should be suspected (Nathan et al., 2021). For diagnosis, a lumbar puncture is required to retrieve the CSF for culture and analysis. The total rate of cultural positivity is more than 80%. Even if additional infections are detected, a positive CSF culture should not be considered a contaminant, especially in immunocompromised individuals (Sánchez–Portocarrero et al., 2000). Furthermore, when Candida spp. is the causative organism, peripheral blood cultures have been considered beneficial (Góralska et al., 2018).

According to a review of the literature, combined Liposomal amphotericin B and flucytosine therapy without intrathecal instillation is the most appropriate therapy for diffused parenchymal infection and meningitis (Nathan et al., 2021). The usual dosage is 3-5 mg/kg of liposomal amphotericin B. Flucytosine is administered at a rate of 25 mg/kg every 6 hours (Pappas et al., 2016). Although drug levels in the cerebrospinal fluid (CSF) and brain are low, amphotericin B is recommended because of its fungicidal effectiveness against basically all Candida species (Groll et al., 2000). Due to emerging resistance, the use of flucytosine monotherapy is limited. Flucytosine administration has been linked to hematologic and liver toxicity. The blood cell count should be carefully monitored. Monitoring the serum concentration of flucytosine in patients with renal dysfunction will be useful for dose adjustment (Vermes et al., 2000).

Fluconazole has strong CNS penetration and is effective against the majority of Candida isolates that cause CNS infections (Johnson and Kauffman, 2003). Fluconazole 400-800 mg (6-12 mg/kg) daily is recommended for step-down treatment once the patient has responded to the starting regimen (Pappas et al., 2016).

Antifungal medication should be continued until all abscesses on magnetic resonance imaging (MRI) have resolved; CSF protein, culture, pleocytosis, and glucose have returned to normal levels; and the patient's symptoms and signs have recovered (Pappas et al., 2016).

Mucormycosis (Zygomycosis)

After aspergillosis, mucormycosis is the second most common invasive mold disease. It is caused by a filamentous fungus of the order Mucorales (Chikley et al., 2019). These fungi are frequently found in soil, compost piles, decaying organic debris, bread, fruits, vegetables, and animal excrement (Ribes et al., 2000). Rhizopus, Mucor, and Lichtheimia species comprise the great majority of Mucorales species that infect people (Nathan et al., 2021). Rhizopus species (47%) and Mucor species (18%) were the most frequent causes of culture-confirmed mucormycosis in a worldwide review of more than 900 mucormycosis cases (Kwon-Chung, 2012; Roden et al., 2005; Gomes et al., 2011).

The predominant route of infection is by inhaling sporangiospores, the asexual spores of Mucorales, which results in invasive sinopulmonary infection. Penetration of CNS occurs by cranial infiltration through the paranasal sinuses or hematogenous spread (Chikley et al., 2019). The invasive fungus may expand laterally into the cavernous sinus to involve the orbits, inferiorly to infiltrate the palate, posteriorly to invade the sphenoid sinus, and cranially to infect the brain (Hosseini and Borghei, 2005). Uncontrolled diabetes mellitus (both type 1 and type 2), metabolic acidosis, high-dose glucocorticoid treatment, penetrating trauma or burns, persistent neutropenia, and deferoxamine chelation treatment in patients who were on dialysis or chronically transfusion dependent are among the most common underlying risk factors for invasive mucormycosis (Roden et al., 2005; Ribes et al., 2000).

In addition to other risk factors, numerous opportunistic diseases, including candidiasis, aspergillosis, and mucormycosis, are more frequently associated with Coronavirus disease 2019 (COVID-19) infections (Nagalli and Kikkeri, 2021). In COVID-19 patients, steroids have probably increased the probability that mucormycosis occurs in diabetic individuals. Steroids raise blood sugar levels, which leads to the glycosylation of ferritin and transferrin, reduces iron binding, and increases the amount of free iron. This helps the germination of mucor spores coupled with the acidity caused by diabetic ketoacidosis. Steroid-induced suppression of leucocyte phagocytic activity is another factor in the pathogenesis of the condition (Singh et al., 2021).

Rhino-orbital-cerebral mucormycosis is the most common clinical presentation of mucormycosis. When mucormycosis affects the sinuses, it initially infects the paranasal sinuses and the turbinates. At this point of the disease, symptoms such as congestion, hyposmia, sinus discomfort, face or mouth pain, and anosmia could be difficult to identify from other more common causes of sinusitis (Mantadakis and Samonis, 2009; Yohai et al., 1994). The nasal mucosa initially becomes erythematous, later becomes a deep purple color, and ultimately black as tissue necrosis begins. Bloody nasal discharge and necrotic eschars on the hard palate or nasal mucosa are sentinel signs that should alert clinicians that mucormycosis may be present (Yohai et al., 1994; Walsh et al., 2014). On the other hand, while necrotic nasal or palatal lesions can only appear in 50% of patients after 3 days of infection, the lack of lesions or necrotic eschars is not enough to rule out the risk of rhinocerebral infection (Bennett et al., 2015, p.2912).

Clinically useful circulating mucormycosis indicators are not yet available (Dadwal and Kontoyiannis, 2018). Hence, microbiological examinations of tissue acquired by biopsy or surgical debridement are necessary for a conclusive diagnosis. By performing a direct microscopic examination on fresh tissue, a preliminary diagnosis can be determined (Schelenz et al., 2015). Thick, hyaline, branching, nonseptate hyphae are visible upon histopathology analysis of fixed and direct preparations of the obtainable biological samples (autopsy material, CSF, surgically resected samples, and biopsy samples) (Góralska et al., 2018).

Early identification, reversion of underlying risk factors, prompt surgical removal of diseased tissue, and prompt beginning of efficient, high-dose systemic antifungal medication are all required for successful treatment of mucormycosis (Bennet et al., 2015, p.2917).

The drug of choice is liposomal amphotericin B, and the dosage should be at least 5 mg/kg/day. It is not recommended to use amphotericin B deoxycholate (Cornerly et al., 2013).

Conclusion

As the prevalence of CNS fungal infections has increased in recent years, so has the awareness of these diseases. The mortality and morbidity rates of the CNS fungal infections, however, remain high. To reduce these rates, a more rapid diagnosis and prompt, effective medical and surgical treatment are needed.

References

Arsura, E. L., Johnson, R., Penrose, J., Stewart, K., Kilgore, W., Reddy, C. M., & Bobba, R. K. (2005). Neuroimaging as a guide to predict outcomes for patients with Coccidioidal meningitis. *Clinical Infectious Diseases*, 40(4), 624-627. https://doi.org/10.1086/427215.

Ashraf, N., Kubat, R. C., Poplin, V., Adenis, A. A., Denning, D. W., Wright, L., McCotter, O., Schwartz, I. S., Jackson, B. R., Chiller, T., & Bahr, N. C. (2020). Re-drawing the maps for endemic mycoses. *Mycopathologia*, 185(5), 843-865. https://doi.org/10.1007/s11046-020-00431-2.

Arastehfar, A., Carvalho, A., Houbraken, J., Lombardi, L., Garcia-Rubio, R., Jenks, J., Rivero-Menendez, O., Aljohani, R., Jacobsen, I., Berman, J., Osherov, N., Hedayati, M., Ilkit, M., Armstrong-James, D., Gabaldón, T., Meletiadis, J., Kostrzewa, M., Pan, W., Lass-Flörl, C., Perlin, D.D., & Hoenigl, M. (2021). Aspergillus fumigatusand aspergillosis: From basics to clinics. *Studies in Mycology*, 100(1), 100115-100115. https://doi.org/10.1016/j.simyco.2021.100115.

Baddley, J., Andes, D., Marr, K., Kontoyiannis, D., Alexander, B., Kauffman, C., Oster, R., Anaissie, E., Walsh, T., Schuster, M., Wingard, J., Patterson, T., Ito, J., Williams, O., Chiller, T., & Pappas, P. (2010). Factors associated with mortality in transplant patients with invasive aspergillosis. *Clinical Infectious Diseases*, 50(12), 1559-1567. https://doi.org/10.1086/652768.

Bariola, J., Perry, P., Pappas, P., Proia, L., Shealey, W., Wright, P., Sizemore, J., Robinson, M., & Bradsher, R. (2010). Blastomycosis of the central nervous system: A multicenter review of diagnosis and treatment in the modern era. *Clinical Infectious Diseases*, 50(6), 797-804. https://doi.org/10.1086/650579.

Barnes, P. D., & Marr, K. A. (2006). Aspergillosis: Spectrum of disease, diagnosis, and treatment. *Infectious Disease Clinics of North America*, 20(3), 545-561. https://doi.org/10.1016/j.idc.2006.06.001.

Ben-Ami, R. (2018). Treatment of invasive candidiasis: A narrative review. *Journal of Fungi*, 4(3), 97. https://doi.org/10.3390/jof4030097.

Bicanic, T., Muzoora, C., Brouwer, A., Meintjes, G., Longley, N., Taseera, K., Rebe, K., Loyse, A., Jarvis, J., Bekker, L., Wood, R., Limmathurotsakul, D., Chierakul, W., Stepniewska, K., White, N., Jaffar, S., & Harrison, T. (2009). Independent association between rate of clearance of infection and clinical outcome of HIV-associated

Cryptococcal meningitis: Analysis of a combined cohort of 262 patients. *Clinical Infectious Diseases*, 49(5), 702-709. https://doi.org/10.1086/604716.

Bloch, K. C., Myint, T., Raymond-Guillen, L., Hage, C. A., Davis, T. E., Wright, P. W., Chow, F. C., Woc-Colburn, L., Khairy, R. N., Street, A. C., Yamamoto, T., Albers, A., & Wheat, L. J. (2017). Improvement in diagnosis of Histoplasma meningitis by combined testing for Histoplasma antigen and immunoglobulin G and immunoglobulin M anti-histoplasma antibody in cerebrospinal fluid. *Clinical Infectious Diseases*, 66(1), 89-94. https://doi.org/10.1093/cid/cix706.

Bloch, K. C., & Bailin, S. S. (2019). Update on fungal infections of the central nervous system. *Current Opinion in Infectious Diseases*, 32(3), 277-284. https://doi.org/10.1097/qco.0000000000000541.

Bozzette, S. A., Larsen, R. A., Chiu, J., Leal, M. A., Jacobsen, J., Rothman, P., Robinson, P., Gilbert, G., McCutchan, J. A., Tilles, J., Leedom, J. M., & Richman, D. D. (1991). A placebo-controlled trial of maintenance therapy with fluconazole after treatment of Cryptococcal meningitis in the acquired immunodeficiency syndrome. *New England Journal of Medicine*, 324(9), 580-584. https://doi.org/10.1056/nejm 199102283240902.

Cadena, J., Thompson, G. R., & Patterson, T. F. (2016). Invasive aspergillosis. *Infectious Disease Clinics of North America*, 30(1), 125-142. https://doi.org/10.1016/ j.idc.2015.10.015.

Candoni, A., Klimko, N., Busca, A., Di Blasi, R., Shadrivova, O., Cesaro, S., Zannier, M. E., Verga, L., Forghieri, F., Calore, E., Nadali, G., Simonetti, E., Muggeo, P., Quinto, A., Castagnola, C., Cellini, M., Del Principe, M., Fracchiolla, N., & Melillo, L. (2019). Fungal infections of the central nervous system and paranasal sinuses in onco-haematologic patients. Epidemiological study reporting the diagnostic-therapeutic approach and outcome in 89 cases. *Mycoses*, 62(3), 252-260. https://doi.org/10.1111/myc.12884.

Casadevall, A., & Perfect, J. R. (1998). *Cryptococcus neoformans*. https://doi.org/10.1128/9781555818241.

Chapman, S. W., Dismukes, W. E., Proia, L. A., Bradsher, R. W., Pappas, P. G., Threlkeld, M. G., & Kauffman, C. A. (2008). Clinical practice guidelines for the management of Blastomycosis: 2008 update by the Infectious Diseases Society of America. *Clinical Infectious Diseases*, 46(12), 1801-1812. https://doi.org/10.1086/588300.

Chayakulkeeree, M., & Perfect, J. R. (2006). Cryptococcosis. *Infectious Disease Clinics of North America*, 20(3), 507-544. https://doi.org/10.1016/j.idc.2006.07.001.

Chikley, A., Ben-Ami, R., & Kontoyiannis. D. P. (2019). Mucormycosis of the central nervous system. *Journal of Fungi*, 5(3), 59. https://doi.org/10.3390/jof5030059.

Chowfin, A., Tight, R., & Mitchell, S. (2000). Recurrent Blastomycosis of the central nervous system: Case report and review. *Clinical Infectious Diseases*, 30(6), 969-971. https://doi.org/10.1086/313828.

Cornely, O. A., Arikan-Akdagli, S., Dannaoui, E., Groll, A. H., Lagrou, K., Chakrabarti, A., Lanternier, F., Pagano, L., Skiada, A., Akova, M., Arendrup, M. C., Boekhout, T., Chowdhary, A., Cuenca-Estrella, M., Freiberger, T., Guinea, J., Guarro, J., de Hoog, S., Hope, W., Johnson, E., Kathuria, S., Lackner, M., Lass-Flörl, C., Lortholary, O., Meis, J.F., Meletiadis, J., Muñoz, P., Richardson, M., Roilides, E., Tortorano, A.M.,

Ullmann, A.J., van Diepeningen, A., Verweij, P., Petrikkos, G. (2014). ESCMID and ECMM joint clinical guidelines for the diagnosis and management of mucormycosis 2013. *Clinical Microbiology and Infection*, 20(3), 5–26. https://doi.org/10.1111/1469-0691.12371.

Clinicalinfo.HIV.gov (2023). Guidelines for the Prevention and Treatment of Opportunistic Infections in Adults and Adolescents with HIV: Cryptococcosis. NIH. (n.d.). Clinicalinfo Information on HIV/AIDS Treatment Prevention and Research. Retrieved from: https://clinicalinfo.hiv.gov/en/guidelines/hiv-clinical-guidelines-adult-and-adolescent-opportunistic-infections/cryptococcosis.

Dadwal, S. S., & Kontoyiannis, D. P. (2018). Recent advances in the molecular diagnosis of mucormycosis. *Expert Review of Molecular Diagnostics*, 18(10), 845-854. https://doi.org/10.1080/14737159.2018.1522250.

Dewsnup, D. H. (1996). Is it ever safe to stop Azole therapy for Coccidioides immitis meningitis?. *Annals of Internal Medicine*, 124(3), 305. https://doi.org/10.7326/0003-4819-124-3-199602010-00004.

De Pauw, B., Walsh, T. J., Donnelly, J. P., Stevens, D. A., Edwards, J. E., Calandra, T., Pappas, P. G., Maertens, J., Lortholary, O., Kauffman, C. A., Denning, D. W., Patterson, T. F., Maschmeyer, G., Bille, J., Dismukes, W. E., Herbrecht, R., Hope, W. W., Kibbler, C. C., Kullberg, B. J., Marr, K. A., Muñoz, P., Odds, F. C., Perfect, J. R., Restrepo, A., Ruhnke, M., Segal, B. H., Sobel, J. D., Sorrell, T. C., Viscoli, C., Wingard, J. R., Zaoutis, T. & Bennett, J. E. (2008). Revised Definitions of Invasive Fungal Disease from the European Organization for Research and Treatment of Cancer/Invasive Fungal Infections Cooperative Group and the National Institute of Allergy and Infectious Diseases Mycoses Study Group (EORTC/MSG) Consensus Group. *Clinical Infectious Diseases*. 1813-21. https://doi.org/10.1086/588660.

Drutz, D. J., & Frey, C. L. (1985). Intracellular and extracellular defenses of human phagocytes against Blastomyces dermatitidis conidia and yeasts. *The Journal of Laboratory and Clinical Medicine*, 105(6), 737–750.

Eichner, R., Al Salami, M., Wood, P., & Müllbacher, A. (1986). The effect of gliotoxin upon macrophage function. *International Journal of Immunopharmacology*, 8(7), 789-797. https://doi.org/10.1016/0192-0561(86)90016-0.

Einstein, H.E., Holeman, C. W., Jr, Sandidge, L. L., and Holden, D. H. (1961). Coccidioidal meningitis. The use of amphotericin B in treatment. *California medicine*, 94(6), 339–343.

Eisenman, H. C., Casadevall, A., & McClelland, E. E. (2007). New insights on the pathogenesis of invasive Cryptococcus neoformans infection. *Current Infectious Disease Reports*, 9(6), 457-464. https://doi.org/10.1007/s11908-007-0070-8.

Forster, J., Hoenigl, M., Suerbaum, S., Wagener, J., & Dichtl, K. (2022). Serologic biomarkers in Candida and Aspergillus infections of the central nervous system: A comparison of galactomannan, mannan and β-1,3-D-glucan testing from serum and cerebrospinal fluid. *Mycoses*, 65(7), 709-714. https://doi.org/10.1111/myc.13451.

Goldstein, E. J., Johnson, R. H., & Einstein, H. E. (2006). Coccidioidal meningitis. *Clinical Infectious Diseases*, 42(1), 103-107. https://doi.org/10.1086/497596.

Gomes, M. Z., Lewis, R. E., & Kontoyiannis, D. P. (2011). Mucormycosis caused by unusual Mucormycetes, non-rhizopus, -mucor, and -lichtheimia species. *Clinical Microbiology Reviews*, 24(2), 411-445. https://doi.org/10.1128/cmr.00056-10.

Goodman, J. S., Kaufman, L., & Koenig, M. G. (1971). Diagnosis of Cryptococcal meningitis. *New England Journal of Medicine*, 285(8), 434-436. https://doi.org/10.1056/nejm197108192850804.

Góralska, K., Blaszkowska, J., & Dzikowiec, M. (2018). Neuroinfections caused by fungi. *Infection*, 46(4), 443-459. https://doi.org/10.1007/s15010-018-1152-2.

Groll, A. H., Giri, N., Petraitis, V., Petraitiene, R., Candelario, M., Bacher, J. S., Piscitelli, S. C., & Walsh, T. J. (2000). Comparative efficacy and distribution of lipid formulations of amphotericin B in experimental Candida albicans infection of the central nervous system. *The Journal of Infectious Diseases*, 182(1), 274–282. https://doi.org/10.1086/315643.

Guidelines for diagnosing, preventing and managing cryptococcal disease among adults, adolescents and children living with HIV. Geneva: World Health Organization; 2022. Licence: CC BY-NC-SA 3.0 IGO.

Harris, J., Lockhart, S., & Chiller, T. (2012). Cryptococcus gattii: Where do we go from here? *Medical Mycology*, 50(2), 113-129. https://doi.org/10.3109/13693786.2011.607854.

Herbrecht, R., Denning, D. W., Patterson, T. F., Bennett, J. E., Greene, R. E., Oestmann, J., Kern, W. V., Marr, K. A., Ribaud, P., Lortholary, O., Sylvester, R., Rubin, R. H., Wingard, J. R., Stark, P., Durand, C., Caillot, D., Thiel, E., Chandrasekar, P. H., Hodges, M. R., Schlamm, H. T., Troke, P. F., & De Pauw, B. (2002). Intracellular and extracellular defenses of human phagocytes against Blastomyces dermatitidis conidia and yeasts. *New England Journal of Medicine*, 347(6), 408-415. https://doi.org/10.1056/nejmoa020191.

Hosseini, S. M., & Borghei, P. (2005). Rhinocerebral mucormycosis: Pathways of spread. *European Archives of Oto-Rhino-Laryngology*, 262(11), 932-938. https://doi.org/10.1007/s00405-005-0919-0.

Jackson, N. R., Blair, J. E., & Ampel, N. M. (2019). Central nervous system infections due to coccidioidomycosis. *Journal of Fungi*, 5(3), 54. https://doi.org/10.3390/jof5030054.

Jenks, J. D., & Hoenigl, M. (2020). Point-of-care diagnostics for invasive aspergillosis: Nearing the finish line. *Expert Review of Molecular Diagnostics*, 20(10), 1009-1017. https://doi.org/10.1080/14737159.2020.1820864.

John, E. B., Raphael, D., Martin, J. B. (2015). *Mandell, Douglas, and Bennett's principles and practice of infectious diseases.* (8th ed.). Philadelphia, PA: Elsevier/Saunders, https://doi.org/10.1016/C2012-1-00075-6.

Johnson, L. B., & Kauffman, C. A. (2003). Voriconazole: a new triazole antifungal agent. *Clinical Infectious Diseases*, 36(5), 630–637. https://doi.org/10.1086/367933.

Johnson, R., Ho, J., Fowler, P., & Heidari, A. (2018). Coccidioidal meningitis: A review on diagnosis, treatment, and management of complications. *Current Neurology and Neuroscience Reports*, 18(4). https://doi.org/10.1007/s11910-018-0824-8.

Kauffman, C. A., Bergman, A. G., Severance, P. J., & McClatchey, K. D. (1981). Detection of Cryptococcal antigen: Comparison of two LaTeX agglutination tests. *American Journal of Clinical Pathology*, 75(1), 106-109. https://doi.org/10.1093/ajcp/75.1.106.

Kauffman, C. A. (2019). Central nervous system infection with other endemic mycoses: Rare manifestation of Blastomycosis, Paracoccidioidomycosis, Talaromycosis, and sporotrichosis. *Journal of Fungi*, 5(3), 64. https://doi.org/10.3390/jof5030064.

Kelly, P. C. (1980). Coccidioidal meningitis. *Coccidioidomycosis*, 163-193. https://doi.org/10.1007/978-1-4757-1712-9_11.

Kirkland, T. N., & Fierer, J. (2018). Coccidioides immitis and posadasii; A review of their biology, genomics, pathogenesis, and host immunity. *Virulence*, 9(1), 1426-1435. https://doi.org/10.1080/21505594.2018.1509667.

Kohler, J. R., Casadevall, A., & Perfect, J. (2014). The spectrum of fungi that infects humans. *Cold Spring Harbor Perspectives in Medicine*, 5(1), a019273-a019273. https://doi.org/10.1101/cshperspect.a019273.

Kourkoumpetis, T. K., Desalermos, A., Muhammed, M., & Mylonakis, E. (2012). Central nervous system aspergillosis. *Medicine*, 91(6), 328-336. https://doi.org/10.1097/md.0b013e318274cd77.

Kwon-Chung, K. J. (2012). Taxonomy of fungi causing Mucormycosis and Entomophthoramycosis (Zygomycosis) and nomenclature of the disease: Molecular mycologic perspectives. *Clinical Infectious Diseases*, 54(suppl_1), S8-S15. https://doi.org/10.1093/cid/cir864.

Lamoth, F. (2016). Galactomannan and 1,3-β-d-Glucan testing for the diagnosis of invasive aspergillosis. *Journal of Fungi*, 2(3), 22. https://doi.org/10.3390/jof2030022.

Leenders, A. C., Reiss, P., Portegies, P., Clezy, K., Hop, W. C., Hoy, J., Borleffs, J. C., Allworth, T., Kauffmann, R. H., Jones, P., Kroon, F. P., Verbrugh, H. A., & De Marie, S. (1997). Liposomal amphotericin B (AmBisome) compared with amphotericin B both followed by oral fluconazole in the treatment of AIDS-associated cryptococcal meningitis. *AIDS*, 11(12), 1463-1471. https://doi.org/10.1097/00002030-199712000-00010.

Lewis, R. E., Wiederhold, N. P., Chi, J., Han, X. Y., Komanduri, K. V., Kontoyiannis, D. P., & Prince, R. A. (2005). Detection of Gliotoxin in experimental and human aspergillosis. *Infection and Immunity*, 73(1), 635-637. https://doi.org/10.1128/iai.73.1.635-637.2005.

Lewis, R. E., Wiederhold, N. P., Lionakis, M. S., Prince, R. A., & Kontoyiannis, D. P. (2005). Frequency and species distribution of gliotoxin-producing Aspergillus isolates recovered from patients at a tertiary-care Cancer Center. *Journal of Clinical Microbiology*, 43(12), 6120-6122. https://doi.org/10.1128/jcm.43.12.6120-6122.2005.

Li, Q., You, C., Liu, Q., & Liu, Y. (2009). Central nervous system cryptococcoma in immunocompetent patients: a short review illustrated by a new case. *Acta Neurochirurgica*, 152(1), 129-136. https://doi.org/10.1007/s00701-009-0311-8.

Linder, K. A., Kauffman, C. A., & Miceli, M. H. (2023). Blastomycosis: A review of mycological and clinical aspects. *Journal of Fungi*, 9(1), 117. https://doi.org/10.3390/jof9010117.

Liu, Y., Mittal, R., Solis, N. V., Prasadarao, N. V., & Filler, S. G. (2011). Mechanisms of candida albicans trafficking to the brain. *PLoS Pathogens*, 7(10), e1002305. https://doi.org/10.1371/journal.ppat.1002305.

Luckowitsch, M., Rudolph, H., Bochennek, K., Porto, L., & Lehrnbecher, T. (2021). Central nervous system mold infections in children with hematological malignancies: Advances in diagnosis and treatment. *Journal of Fungi*, 7(3), 168. https://doi.org/10.3390/jof7030168.

McBride, J. A., Gauthier, G. M., & Klein, B. S. (2017). Clinical manifestations and treatment of Blastomycosis. *Clinics in Chest Medicine*, 38(3), 435-449. https://doi.org/10.1016/j.ccm.2017.04.006

Maertens, J. A., Raad, I. I., Marr, K. A., Patterson, T. F., Kontoyiannis, D. P., Cornely, O. A., Bow, E. J., Rahav, G., Neofytos, D., Aoun, M., Baddley, J. W., Giladi, M., Heinz, W. J., Herbrecht, R., Hope, W., Karthaus, M., Lee, D. G., Lortholary, O., Morrison, V. A., Oren, I., Selleslag D., A. J. Shoham S., Thompson 3rd G. R., Lee M., Maher R. M., Schmidt-Hoffmann A. H., Zeiher B., & Ullmann, A. J. (2016). Isavuconazole versus voriconazole for primary treatment of invasive mould disease caused by Aspergillus and other filamentous fungi (SECURE): a phase 3, randomised-controlled, non-inferiority trial. *The Lancet*, 387(10020), 760–769. https://doi.org/10.1016/S0140-6736(15)01159-9.

Maertens, J. A., Rahav, G., Lee, D. G., Ponce-de-León, A., Ramírez Sánchez, I. C., Klimko, N., Sonet, A., Haider, S., Diego Vélez, J., Raad, I., Koh, L. P., Karthaus, M., Zhou, J., Ben-Ami, R., Motyl, M. R., Han, S., Grandhi, A., Waskin, H., & study investigators (2021). Posaconazole versus voriconazole for primary treatment of invasive aspergillosis: a phase 3, randomised, controlled, non-inferiority trial. *The Lancet*, 397(10273), 499–509. https://doi.org/10.1016/S0140-6736(21)00219-1.

Magill, S. S., Edwards, J. R., Bamberg, W., Beldavs, Z. G., Dumyati, G., Kainer, M. A., Lynfield, R., Maloney, M., McAllister-Hollod, L., Nadle, J., Ray, S. M., Thompson, D. L., Wilson, L. E., & Fridkin, S. K. (2014). Multistate point-prevalence survey of health care–associated infections. *New England Journal of Medicine*, 370(13), 1198-1208. https://doi.org/10.1056/nejmoa1306801.

Mantadakis, E., & Samonis, G. (2009). Clinical presentation of zygomycosis. *Clinical Microbiology and Infection*, 15, 15-20. https://doi.org/10.1111/j.1469-0691.2009.02974.x.

McCarthy, M., Rosengart, A., Schuetz, A. N., Kontoyiannis, D. P., & Walsh, T. J. (2014). Mold infections of the central nervous system. *New England Journal of Medicine*, 371(2), 150-160. https://doi.org/10.1056/nejmra1216008.

Miceli, M. H. (2019). Central nervous system infections due to aspergillus and other hyaline molds. *Journal of Fungi*, 5(3), 79. https://doi.org/10.3390/jof5030079.

Mikulska, M., Furfaro, E., Del Bono, V., Raiola, A. M., Di Grazia, C., Bacigalupo, A., & Viscoli, C. (2013). (1-3)-β-D-Glucan in cerebrospinal fluid is useful for the diagnosis of central nervous system fungal infections. *Clinical Infectious Diseases*, 56(10), 1511-1512. https://doi.org/10.1093/cid/cit073.

Mousavi, B., Hedayati, M. T., Hedayati, N., Ilkit, M., & Syedmousavi, S. (2016). Aspergillus species in indoor environments and their possible occupational and public health hazards. *Current Medical Mycology*, 2(1), 36-42. https://doi.org/10.18869/acadpub.cmm.2.1.36.

Murayama, T., Amitani, R., Ikegami, Y., Nawada, R., Lee, W., & Kuze, F. (1996). Suppressive effects of aspergillus fumigatus culture filtrates on human alveolar macrophages and polymorphonuclear leucocytes. *European Respiratory Journal*, 9(2), 293-300. https://doi.org/10.1183/09031936.96.09020293.

Murthy, J., & Sundaram, C. (2014). Fungal infections of the central nervous system. *Handbook of Clinical Neurology*, 1383-1401. https://doi.org/10.1016/b978-0-7020-4088-7.00095-x.

Mwaba, P., Mwansa, J., Chintu, C., Pobee, J., Scarborough, M., Portsmouth, S., & Zumla, A. (2001). Clinical presentation, natural history, and cumulative death rates of 230 adults with primary cryptococcal meningitis in zambian AIDS patients treated under local conditions. *Postgraduate Medical Journal*, 77(914), 769-773. https://doi.org/10.1136/pgmj.77.914.769.

Nadkarni, T., & Goel, A. (2005). Aspergilloma of the brain: an overview. *Journal of Postgraduate Medicine*, 51 Suppl 1, S37–S41.

Nagalli, S., & Kikkeri, N. S. (2021). Mucormycosis in COVID-19: A systematic review of literature. *Infezioni in Medicina*, 29(4), 504-512. https://doi.org/10.53854/liim-2904-2.

Nathan, C. L., Emmert, B. E., Nelson, E., & Berger, J. R. (2021). CNS fungal infections: A review. *Journal of the Neurological Sciences*, 422, 117325. https://doi.org/10.1016/j.jns.2021.117325.

Panackal, A. A., & Williamson, P. R. (2015). Fungal infections of the central nervous system. *CONTINUUM: Lifelong Learning in Neurology*, 21, 1662-1678. https://doi.org/10.1212/con.0000000000000241.

Panicker, J., Walsh, T., & Kamani, N. (2006). Recurrent central nervous system blastomycosis in an immunocompetent child treated successfully with sequential liposomal amphotericin B and voriconazole. *The Pediatric Infectious Disease Journal*, 25(4), 377–379. https://doi.org/10.1097/01.inf.0000207475.89745.51.

Pappas, P., Chetchotisakd, P., Larsen, R., Manosuthi, W., Morris, M., Anekthananon, T., Sungkanuparph, S., Supparatpinyo, K., Nolen, T., Zimmer, L., Kendrick, A., Johnson, P., Sobel, J., & Filler, S. (2009). A phase II randomized trial of Amphotericin B alone or combined with fluconazole in the treatment of HIV-associated Cryptococcal meningitis. *Clinical Infectious Diseases*, 48(12), 1775-1783. https://doi.org/10.1086/599112.

Pappas, P. G. (2011). Candidemia in the intensive care unit: Miles to go before we sleep. *Critical Care Medicine*, 39(4), 884-885. https://doi.org/10.1097/ccm.0b013e31820f710b.

Pappas, P. G., Kauffman, C. A., Andes, D. R., Clancy, C. J., Marr, K. A., Ostrosky-Zeichner, L., Reboli, A. C., Schuster, M. G., Vazquez, J. A., Walsh, T. J., Zaoutis, T. E., & Sobel, J. D. (2016). Clinical Practice Guideline for the Management of Candidiasis: 2016 Update by the Infectious Diseases Society of America. *Clinical Infectious Disease*, 62(4), e1–e50. https://doi.org/10.1093/cid/civ933.

Pappas, P. G., Lionakis, M. S., Arendrup, M. C., Ostrosky-Zeichner, L., & Kullberg, B. J. (2018). Invasive candidiasis. *Nature Reviews Disease Primers*, 4(1). https://doi.org/10.1038/nrdp.2018.26.

Park, B. J., Wannemuehler, K. A., Marston, B. J., Govender, N., Pappas, P. G., & Chiller, T. M. (2009). Estimation of the current global burden of cryptococcal meningitis among persons living with HIV/AIDS. *AIDS*, 23(4), 525-530. https://doi.org/10.1097/qad.0b013e328322ffac.

Pascual, A., Csajka, C., Buclin, T., Bolay, S., Bille, J., Calandra, T., & Marchetti, O. (2012). Challenging recommended oral and intravenous Voriconazole doses for improved efficacy and safety: Population pharmacokinetics–based analysis of adult patients with invasive fungal infections. *Clinical Infectious Diseases*, 55(3), 381-390. https://doi.org/10.1093/cid/cis437.

Patterson, T. F., Kirkpatrick, W. R., White, M., Hiemenz, J. W., Wingard, J. R., Dupont, B., Rinaldi, M. G., Stevens, D. A., & Graybill, J. R. (2000). Invasive aspergillosis disease spectrum, treatment practices, and outcomes. *Medicine*, 79(4), 250-260. https://doi.org/10.1097/00005792-200007000-00006.

Patterson, T. F., Thompson, G. R., Denning, D. W., Fishman, J. A., Hadley, S., Herbrecht, R., Kontoyiannis, D. P., Marr, K. A., Morrison, V. A., Nguyen, M. H., Segal, B. H., Steinbach, W. J., Stevens, D. A., Walsh, T. J., Wingard, J. R., Young, J. H., & Bennett, J. E. (2016). Practice guidelines for the diagnosis and management of aspergillosis: 2016 update by the Infectious Diseases Society of America. *Clinical Infectious Diseases*, 63(4), e1-e60. https://doi.org/10.1093/cid/ciw326.

Perfect, J. R., Durack, D. T. and Gallis, H. A. (1983). Cryptococcemia. *Medicine*, 62(2), 98-109. https://doi.org/10.1097/00005792-198303000-00003.

Perfect, J. R. (1989). Cryptococcosis. *Infectious Disease Clinics of North America*, 3(1), 77-102. https://doi.org/10.1016/s0891-5520(20)30248-8.

Pfaller, M. A., & Diekema, D. J. (2007). Epidemiology of invasive candidiasis: A persistent public health problem. *Clinical Microbiology Reviews*, 20(1), 133-163. https://doi.org/10.1128/cmr.00029-06.

Plum, F. (1977). Handbook of clinical neurology edited by P. J. Vinken and G. W. Bruyn, North Holland publishing company. Amsterdam. *Annals of Neurology*, 1(1), 110-110. https://doi.org/10.1002/ana.410010114.

Poplin, V., Smith, C., Milsap, D., Zabel, L., & Bahr, N. C. (2021). Diagnosis of pulmonary infections due to endemic fungi. *Diagnostics*, 11(5), 856. https://doi.org/10.3390/diagnostics11050856.

Pullen, M. F., Alpern, J. D., & Bahr, N. C. (2022). Blastomycosis—Some progress but still much to learn. *Journal of Fungi*, 8(8), 824. https://doi.org/10.3390/jof8080824.

Raman Sharma, R. (2010). Fungal infections of the nervous system: Current perspective and controversies in management. *International Journal of Surgery*, 8(8), 591-601. https://doi.org/10.1016/j.ijsu.2010.07.293.

Ribes, J. A., Vanover-Sams, C. L., & Baker, D. J. (2000). Zygomycetes in human disease. *Clinical Microbiology Reviews*, 13(2), 236-301. https://doi.org/10.1128/cmr.13.2.236.

Riddell, J., & Wheat, L. J. (2019). Central nervous system infection with Histoplasma capsulatum. *Journal of Fungi*, 5(3), 70. https://doi.org/10.3390/jof5030070.

Roden, M. M., Zaoutis, T. E., Buchanan, W. L., Knudsen, T. A., Sarkisova, T. A., Schaufele, R. L., Sein, M., Sein, T., Chiou, C. C., Chu, J. H., Kontoyiannis, D. P., & Walsh, T. J. (2005). Epidemiology and outcome of Zygomycosis: A review of 929 reported cases. *Clinical Infectious Diseases*, 41(5), 634-653. https://doi.org/10.1086/432579.

Ruhnke, M., Kofla, G., Otto, K., & Schwartz, S. (2007). CNS aspergillosis. *CNS Drugs*, 21(8), 659-676. https://doi.org/10.2165/00023210-200721080-00004.

Saccente, M., & Woods, G. L. (2010). Clinical and laboratory update on Blastomycosis. *Clinical Microbiology Reviews*, 23(2), 367-381. https://doi.org/10.1128/cmr.00056-09.

Safdar A. (2013). Immunotherapy for invasive mold disease in severely immunosuppressed patients. *Clinical infectious diseases: an official publication of the Infectious Diseases Society of America*, 57(1), 94–100. https://doi.org/10.1093/cid/cit187.

Sánchez–Portocarrero, J., Pérez–Cecilia, E., Corral, O., Romero–Vivas, J., & Picazo, J. J. (2000). The central nervous system and infection by candida species. *Diagnostic Microbiology and Infectious Disease*, 37(3), 169-179. https://doi.org/10.1016/s0732-8893(00)00140-1.

Schelenz, S., Barnes, R. A., Barton, R. C., Cleverley, J. R., Lucas, S. B., Kibbler, C. C., & Denning, D. W. (2015). British society for medical mycology best practice recommendations for the diagnosis of serious fungal diseases. *The Lancet Infectious Diseases*, 15(4), 461-474. https://doi.org/10.1016/s1473-3099(15)70006-x.

Schwartz, S., Ruhnke, M., Ribaud, P., Reed, E., Troke, P., & Thiel, E. (2007). Poor efficacy of amphotericin B-based therapy in CNS aspergillosis. *Mycoses*, 50(3), 196-200. https://doi.org/10.1111/j.1439-0507.2007.01345.x.

Schwartz, S., & Thiel, E. (2009). Cerebral aspergillosis: Tissue penetration is the key. *Medical Mycology*, 47(s1), S387-S393. https://doi.org/10.1080/13693780802537953.

Segal, B. H. (2009). Aspergillosis. *New England Journal of Medicine*, 360(18), 1870-1884. https://doi.org/10.1056/nejmra0808853.

Singh, N., Gayowski, T., Wagener, M. M., Doyle, H., & Marino, I. R. (1997). Invasive fungal infections in liver transplant recipients receiving Tacrolimus as the primary immunosuppressive agent. *Clinical Infectious Diseases*, 24(2), 179-184. https://doi.org/10.1093/clinids/24.2.179.

Singh, A. K., Singh, R., Joshi, S. R., & Misra, A. (2021). Mucormycosis in COVID-19: A systematic review of cases reported worldwide and in India. Diabetes & Metabolic Syndrome: *Clinical Research & Reviews*, 15(4). https://doi.org/10.1016/j.dsx.2021.05.019.

Sipsas, N. V., & Kontoyiannis, D. P. (2006). Clinical issues regarding relapsing aspergillosis and the efficacy of secondary antifungal prophylaxis in patients with hematological malignancies. *Clinical infectious diseases: an official publication of the Infectious Diseases Society of America*, 42(11), 1584–1591. https://doi.org/10.1086/503844.

Smith, J. A., & Kauffman, C. A. (2010). Blastomycosis. *Proceedings of the American Thoracic Society*, 7(3), 173-180. https://doi.org/10.1513/pats.200906-040al.

Soeffker, G., Wichmann, D., Loderstaedt, U., Sobottka, I., Deuse, T., & Kluge, S. (2013). Aspergillus Galactomannan antigen for diagnosis and treatment monitoring in cerebral aspergillosis. *Progress in Transplantation*, 23(1), 71-74. https://doi.org/10.7182/pit2013386.

Stamm, A. M., Diasio, R. B., Dismukes, W. E., Shadomy, S., Cloud, G. A., Bowles, C. A., Karam, G. H., & Espinel-Ingroff, A. (1987). Toxicity of amphotericin B plus flucytosine in 194 patients with cryptococcal meningitis. *The American Journal of Medicine*, 83(2), 236-242. https://doi.org/10.1016/0002-9343(87)90691-7.

Starkey, J., Moritani, T., & Kirby, P. (2014). MRI of CNS fungal infections: Review of aspergillosis to histoplasmosis and everything in between. *Clinical Neuroradiology*, 24(3), 217-230. https://doi.org/10.1007/s00062-014-0305-7.

Stevens, D. (2001). Intrathecal amphotericin in the management of coccidioidal meningitis1. *Seminars in Respiratory Infections*, 16(4), 263-269. https://doi.org/10.1053/srin.2001.29298.

Sun, S., Sekhon, S., & Huppert, M. (1979). Electron microscopic studies of saprobic and parasitic forms of Coccidioides immitis. *Medical Mycology*, 17(3), 265-273. https://doi.org/10.1080/00362177985380391.

Thompson, G. R., Barker, B. M., & Wiederhold, N. P. (2017). Large-scale evaluation of In Vitro Amphotericin B, Triazole, and Echinocandin activity against Coccidioides species from U.S. institutions. *Antimicrobial Agents and Chemotherapy*, 61(4). https://doi.org/10.1128/aac.02634-16.

Tortorano, A. M., Esposto, M. C., Prigitano, A., Grancini, A., Ossi, C., Cavanna, C., & Cascio, G. L. (2012). Cross-reactivity of Fusarium spp. in the aspergillus Galactomannan enzyme-linked Immunosorbent assay. *Journal of Clinical Microbiology*, 50(3), 1051-1053. https://doi.org/10.1128/jcm.05946-11.

Trifilio, S., Pennick, G., Pi, J., Zook, J., Golf, M., Kaniecki, K., Singhal, S., Williams, S., Winter, J., Tallman, M., Gordon, L., Frankfurt, O., Evens, A., & Mehta, J. (2007). Monitoring plasma voriconazole levels may be necessary to avoid subtherapeutic levels in hematopoietic stem cell transplant recipients. *Cancer*, 109(8), 1532-1535. https://doi.org/10.1002/cncr.22568.

UpToDate, (2022). Treatment and prevention of invasive aspergillosis. Retrieved from: https://www.uptodate.com/contents/treatment-and-prevention-of-invasive-aspergillosis.

Vela-Duarte, D., Nyberg, E., Sillau, S., Pate, A., Castellanos, P., Chastain, D. B., Franco-Paredes, C., & Henao-Martínez, A. F. (2019). Lacunar stroke in Cryptococcal meningitis: Clinical and radiographic features. *Journal of Stroke and Cerebrovascular Diseases*, 28(6), 1767-1772. https://doi.org/10.1016/j.jstrokecerebrovasdis.2018.12.043.

Velamakanni, S. S., Bahr, N. C., Musubire, A. K., Boulware, D. R., Rhein, J., & Nabeta, H. W. (2014). Central nervous system cryptococcoma in a ugandan patient with human immunodeficiency virus. *Medical Mycology Case Reports*, 6, 10-13. https://doi.org/10.1016/j.mmcr.2014.08.003.

Vermes, A., Van der Sijs, H., & Guchelaar, H. (2000). Flucytosine: Correlation between toxicity and pharmacokinetic parameters. *Chemotherapy*, 46(2), 86-94. https://doi.org/10.1159/000007260.

Vincent, T., Galgiani, J. N., Huppert, M., & Salkin, D. (1993). The natural history of Coccidioidal meningitis: Va--armed forces cooperative studies, 1955-1958. *Clinical Infectious Diseases*, 16(2), 247-254. https://doi.org/10.1093/clind/16.2.247.

Walsh, T. J., Hier, D. B., & Caplan, L. R. (1985). Aspergillosis of the central nervous system: Clinicopathological analysis of 17 patients. *Annals of Neurology*, 18(5), 574-582. https://doi.org/10.1002/ana.410180511.

Walsh, T. J. (1998). Editorial response: Primary cutaneous aspergillosis--an emerging infection among Immunocompromised patients. *Clinical Infectious Diseases*, 27(3), 453-457. https://doi.org/10.1086/514718.

Walsh, T. J., Anaissie, E. J., Denning, D. W., Herbrecht, R., Kontoyiannis, D. P., Marr, K. A., Morrison, V. A., Segal, B. H., Steinbach, W. J., Stevens, D. A., Van Burik, J., Wingard, J. R., & Patterson, T. F. (2008). *Clinical Infectious Diseases*, 46(3), 327-360. https://doi.org/10.1086/525258.

Walsh, T. J., Skiada, A., Cornely, O. A., Roilides, E., Ibrahim, A., Zaoutis, T., Groll, A., Lortholary, O., Kontoyiannis, D. P., & Petrikkos, G. (2014). Development of new strategies for early diagnosis of mucormycosis from bench to bedside. *Mycoses*, 57, 2-7. https://doi.org/10.1111/myc.12249.

Wheat, L. J., Batteiger, B. E., & Sathapatayavavongs, B. (1990). Histoplasma capsulatum infections of the central nervous system. *Medicine*, 69(4), 244. https://doi.org/10.1097/00005792-199007000-00006.

Wheat, L. J., Freifeld, A. G., Kleiman, M. B., Baddley, J. W., McKinsey, D. S., Loyd, J. E., & Kauffman, C. A. (2007). Clinical practice guidelines for the management of patients with histoplasmosis: 2007 update by the Infectious Diseases Society of America. *Clinical Infectious Diseases*, 45(7), 807-825. https://doi.org/10.1086/521259.

Wheat, J., Myint, T., Guo, Y., Kemmer, P., Hage, C., Terry, C., Azar, M. M., Riddell, J., Ender, P., Chen, S., Shehab, K., Cleveland, K., Esguerra, E., Johnson, J., Wright, P., Douglas, V., Vergidis, P., Ooi, W., Baddley, J., Bamberger D., Khairy D., Vikram H., Jenny-Avital H., Sivasubramanian G., Bowlware K., Pahud B., Sarria J., Tsai T., Assi M., Mocherla S., Prakash V., Allen D., Passaretti C., Huprikar S., & Anderson, A. (2018). Central nervous system histoplasmosis. *Medicine*, 97(13), e0245. https://doi.org/10.1097/md.0000000000010245.

Woods, M., Redmond, A., & Dancer, C. (2007). Fungal infections of the central nervous system: A review of fungal pathogens and treatment. *Neurology India*, 55(3), 251. https://doi.org/10.4103/0028-3886.35686.

Yohai, R. A., Bullock, J. D., Aziz, A. A., & Markert, R. J. (1994). Survival factors in rhino-orbital-cerebral mucormycosis. *Survey of Ophthalmology*, 39(1), 3-22. https://doi.org/10.1016/s0039-6257(05)80041-4.

Chapter 16

Prion Disease

Murat Özsaraç*, **MD**
Department of Emergency Medicine, Sakarya University Faculty of Medicine, Sakarya, Turkiye

Abstract

A prion is a proteinaceous infectious particle. It is a rare, fatal, and extremely rapidly progressive neurodegenerative disease caused by misfolding of the prion protein (PrP). It affects both humans and animals. It may be sporadic, inherited, or acquired through iatrogenic or dietary exposure. It progresses to death within an average of six months to one year after developing symptoms. The symptoms are highly diverse; therefore, clinicians need a low threshold for the diagnosis of prion, although classical presentations are usually easy to diagnose. Diagnostic tools include magnetic resonance imaging, electroencephalogram, and non-specific fluid biomarkers of neuronal damage. The extensive spongy change in the brain is pathognomonic. Abnormal hyperintensity in the cortical gyrus, caudate, putamen, or thalamus is observed with diffusion-weighted imaging (DWI). Currently, there is no effective treatment method. However, a better understanding of the pathogenesis will enable the implementation of effective therapeutic interventions shortly.

Keywords: prion disease, transmissible spongiform encephalopathies, neuroinflammation, microglial activation, astrogliosis, neurodegenerative disease

---

* Corresponding Author's Email: muratozsarac@sakarya.edu.tr.

In: Central Nervous System Infections
Editor: Mustafa Usanmaz
ISBN: 979-8-89113-660-1

Introduction

Prion, a proteinaceous infectious particle, is formed primarily when misfolding transforms the protein with a β-sheet structure into an abnormal form. The standard cellular protein PrP is converted to PrPSc. Particles composed of the modified protein (PrPSc) without nucleic acids are highly contagious. Its conversion to PrPSc is thought to occur spontaneously (or possibly by mutation of PRNP) (Prusiner, 1998).

In genetic prion diseases, mutations in the prion protein gene increase susceptibility to misfolding. Genetic prion diseases caused by mutations in the protein gene (PRNP) are classified according to clinical phenotype, mutation, and neuropathological features. Prion diseases caused by abnormal proteins called Jakob-Creutzfeldt disease if it is sporadic, fatal familial insomnia, Gerstmann-Sträussler-Scheinker syndrome, Jakob-Creutzfeldt disease if genetic, and kuru disease if acquired (Geschwind, 2015). Neuropathology is a similar characteristic in all prionoses. Common underlying molecular mechanisms are neuronal loss, astrogliosis, and characteristic diffuse spongiform encephalopathy, microglial activation, and PrPS Sc accumulation affecting the gray matter of the central nervous system. Besides these, intraneuronal vacuolation, cerebellar plaques, and amyloid deposition are observed in the cerebellum and cerebral hemispheres. Another distinctive histopathological feature is clustered prion protein deposits of varying sizes ranging from soluble, unbranched, small oligomers to long, thin fibrils (Sigurdson, 2019). Although much has been discovered about the mechanisms of prion transformation, transmission, and pathogenesis in recent years, fundamental structural and mechanistic questions in prion diseases remain unresolved. Therefore, it is thought that elucidating the processes related to differences in the structure of PrPSc molecules, the spread of prions in the brain, changes in neural target cells, prion-induced neuronal toxicity, and prion clearance pathways may be a guide in dementia research in recent years (Geschwind, 2015). Sporadic JCD is the most common form of prion disease. Eating contaminated meat products is one of the most critical areas of contamination. Supplementing dairy cow diets with meat and bone products may increase the development chance of the disease. Cases of accidental occupational exposure and further iatrogenic JCD have been reported. It has been demonstrated that transfection may occur due to human-derived growth hormone, human pituitary-derived gonadotropin use, corneal transplants, dura mater grafts, spinal and cerebral surgical instruments, and blood transfusion.

Familial forms of prion disease are autosomally dominant and related to PrP gene mutations (Takada, 2013).

Clinical Picture and Physical Examination

Physical Examination

Clinical symptoms and physical findings vary according to the type of prion disease. The most common initial symptoms are cerebellar dysfunction, ataxia, and cognitive impairment.

Jakob-Creutzfeldt Disease

Cortical dysfunction, visual and behavioral abnormalities, and pyramidal and extrapyramidal symptoms are primarily in the picture. In sporadic CJD, global cognitive impairments, cerebellar dysfunction, myoclonic convulsions, peripheral neuropathy, visual impairment, rapidly progressive multifocal neurologic dysfunction, and clinical findings of akinetic mutism are observed, which progress to the terminal stage and death within eight months. The clinical picture is thought to be caused by the accumulation of PrP(Sc). In addition, patients develop myoclonic convulsions involving the whole body or a limb, which may be exacerbated by auditory or tactile stimulation (Cazzaniga, 2021).

Gerstmann-Straussler-Scheinker Disease

It is diagnosed with neuropathological findings rather than clinical manifestations. There is a family history in 70-100% of patients, and it is autosomal dominant and is caused by mutations of the PrP gene. Brain stem involvement is distinctive. Slowly progressive extremity and truncal ataxia, cognitive decline, psychiatric symptoms, myoclonus, Parkinsonism, and dementia clinics are prominently observed. Death occurs 3-8 years after symptoms begin. It is neuropathologically characterized by the presence of multicentric PrPSc amyloid plaques. This variant of prionoses links the pathogenesis of Alzheimer's disease and prion-related diseases (Kim, 2018).

Fatal Familial Insomnia

It is observed at a very high incidence rate in Spain. The age of onset is variable, between 18-60 years. It manifests itself with dementia, neuro-ophthalmological abnormalities, progressive sympathetic symptoms, dysautonomia (excessive sweating, tachypnea, hypertension, tachycardia, hyperthermia), weight loss, persistent insomnia (Agrypnia excitata), restlessness in sleep, hypnic jumps, twitching in extremities, psychiatric symptoms, catatonia, repetition of simple stereotypical activities of daily living and motor paralysis. The clinical presentations are varied. Genotyping is the gold standard for a definitive diagnosis. It is associated with the D178N mutation of the PRNP gene located on chromosome 20. Significant brain atrophy occurs due to gliosis and neuronal loss in the anterior ventral and mediodorsal thalamic nuclei. Unlike other prionoses, spongy changes are almost absent. The cortex is preserved, but the thalamus is severely damaged (Chu, 2022).

Differential Diagnosis

Prion disease progresses with a highly rapid clinical course. It progresses to death about six months after the first symptoms develop. In genetic prion cases, death occurs within one year from the first symptoms. Patients typically present with rapidly progressive dementia and akinetic mutism in their last weeks. Diagnosis is difficult due to the heterogeneity of early neurocognitive, motor, autonomic, or psychiatric symptoms. Most patients are not diagnosed until two-thirds of the symptomatic course. As a result, patients are often misdiagnosed as having peripheral neuropathy, vasculitis, unspecified dementia, stroke, Alzheimer's disease, dizziness, depression, paraneoplastic disorder, and viral encephalitis (Paterson, 2012). Because Jakob-Creutzfeldt's disease simultaneously affects multiple areas of the brain, its clinical presentation is variable and mimics many other neurological or psychiatric conditions, especially in the early stages. As a result, patients usually receive a different diagnosis about two-thirds of the disease course before a correct diagnosis is made. This is why Jakob-Creutzfeldt's disease is called the "great imitator" (Geschwind, 2015) (Table 1).

Table 1. CDC's diagnostic criteria for Jakob-Creutzfeldt- Disease (JCD)

1. Sporadic CJD *Definite:* Diagnosed by standard neuropathological techniques; and/or immunocytochemically; and/or Western blot confirmed protease-resistant PrP; and /or presence of scrapie-associated fibrils. *Probable:* Neuropsychiatric disorder plus positive RT-QuIC in cerebrospinal fluid (CSF) or other tissues *OR* rapidly progressive dementia; *and* at least two out of the following four clinical features: Myoclonus, Visual or cerebellar signs, Pyramidal/extrapyramidal signs, Akinetic mutism *AND* a positive result on at least one of the following laboratory tests: • a typical EEG (periodic sharp wave complexes) during an illness of any duration • a positive 14-3-3 CSF assay in patients with a disease duration of less than 2 years • High signal in the caudate/putamen on magnetic resonance imaging (MRI) brain scan or at least two cortical regions (temporal, parietal, occipital) either on diffusion-weighted imaging (DWI) or fluid attenuated inversion recovery (FLAIR) *AND* without routine investigations indicating an alternative diagnosis. *Possible:* Progressive dementia; *and* at least two out of the following four clinical features: Myoclonus, Visual or cerebellar signs, Pyramidal/extrapyramidal signs, Akinetic mutism *AND* the absence of a positive result for any of the four tests above that would classify a case as "probable" *AND* duration of illness less than two years *AND* without routine investigations indicating an alternative diagnosis.
2. Iatrogenic CJD: Progressive cerebellar syndrome in a recipient of human cadaveric-derived pituitary hormone; or sporadic CJD with a recognized exposure risk, e.g., antecedent neurosurgery with dura mater implantation.
3. Familial CJD: Definite or probable CJD *plus* definite or probable CJD in a first-degree relative; and/or neuropsychiatric disorder *plus* disease-specific PrP gene mutation.

Zerr, 1998.

Diagnostic Studies

The gold standard method for confirming the diagnosis of sporadic or acquired prion disease, histological examination of brain tissue includes immunohistochemistry and Western blot techniques. Classical neuropathological findings (spongiosis, neuronal loss, PrP accumulation, and gliosis) can be detected with the tests mentioned above (Budka, 1995). With the widespread use of non-invasive examination methods, brain biopsy is performed much less frequently in patients suspected of having prion disease. There are no methods to identify patients with sporadic prion disease before clinical symptoms appear. However, it is stated that although there is a theory that screening individuals with high penetration PRNP mutations with some specific genetic tests can detect the disease years before symptom onset, this is not possible in practice (Vallabh, 2020). One of the greatest challenges in identifying preclinical prion disease is the need for robust preclinical screening methods. Diagnosis of the disease is often delayed unless the patient is evaluated by a clinician familiar with the symptoms of prion. Identifying infectivity and replication early in the disease process has also been a significant hurdle in the development of treatment. New techniques such as Protein Misfolding Cyclic Amplification (PMCA) and Real-Time Quaking Induced Conversion – Real-Time Shake Induced Conversion (RT-QuIC) can be helpful in overcoming this problem. The aggregation of misfolded PrP can be monitored in real-time using fluorescent dyes (Moda, 2019). MRI with DWI and real-time quaking-induced conversion of cerebrospinal fluid (CSF) (RT-QuIC) have emerged as reliable tests. Early diagnosis is essential for the treatment of prion diseases. Characteristic brain MRI lesions help to make the diagnosis. The basal ganglia and cortical hyperintensities are the most common MRI findings (Geschwind et al., 2009). CSF obtained by lumbar puncture has become the primary fluid analyte for the identification of biomarkers in human prion diseases. With the rapidly developing neurodegeneration due to prion disease, it causes an increase in blood markers reflecting axonal neuronal, synaptic, or glial pathology, such as neurofilament light chain, glial fibrillary acidic protein, total tau protein, neuron-specific enolase (NSE), S100β and 14-3-3. However, these tests are not prion specific and do not identify prions. It is stated that such tests, applied together with diagnostic biomarkers, can be predictors of the course of the disease and early detection of asymptomatic individuals at high risk for prion disease in terms of neuronal damage (Forner, 2015). Measuring of the total amount of tau, α-synuclein, and neurofilament light chain in serum using standard ELISA methods by taking blood samples other than CSF may be diagnostically helpful (Thompson, 2019). The use of CSF biomarkers to diagnose sporadic Jakob-Creutzfeldt disease is controversial. A CSF examination is recommended when there is a strong suspicion of the disease, and the diagnosis is still uncertain (Muayqil, 2012).

Imaging Studies

MRI is a diagnostically important imaging assay as it is easily accessible and non-invasive. Diffusion MRI has high diagnostic specificity. Hyperintense signals can be seen in the cortical strip, basal ganglia, and thalamus on diffusion-weighted images (DWI) and (FLAIR) images. Specifically identified radiological findings: the "hockey stick" sign, which corresponds to an increased signal resembling a hockey stick in the head of the caudate nucleus and the putamen, and the "pulvinar" sign, which corresponds to a bilaterally increased signal in the pulvinar thalamic nuclei, are typical for JCD (Bizzi, 2020).

Other Tests

EEG

It may show non-specific abnormalities in the early stages of the disease. The general sensitivity of EEG varies between 40-70%. Repeated recordings show periodic EEG abnormalities in more than 90% of patients. Periodic, three-phase strong wave complexes are pretty typical. During the course of sporadic JCD, most patients develop a characteristic EEG finding with pseudoperiodic paroxysms or periodic spikes or strong waves on a slow background (Mundlamurri, 2020).

Sleep Studies

In cases where sporadic fatal insomnia is suspected, video-polysomnography may be helpful to confirm that total sleep time is significantly reduced or irregular sleep (Abu-Rumeileh, 2018).

Genetic Tests

Although not yet routine, specific tests are performed to determine the genetic risk associated with prionoses. Evaluation of genetic risk determination for the SNP in STX6 in sporadic human prion disease involving sphingolipid metabolism shares a similar causal mechanism with progressive supranuclear palsy, a neurodegenerative disease associated with misfolding of the tau protein (Jones, 2020).

Treatment

All prion diseases are fatal, and patients are currently treated with symptomatic therapies. Currently, there is no effective treatment; however, a better understanding of their pathogenesis has led to the promise of effective therapeutic interventions shortly. Antiepileptics for patients with seizures and anti-Parkinsonian drugs for extrapyramidal symptoms should be given. Prion diseases can be transmitted transcutaneously, peripherally, orally, or hematogenously. In pathogenesis, it has been observed that critical processes in the early stages before neuroinvasion occur outside the nervous system, especially in peripheral lymphoid organs. Inhibition of PrP conversion with early detection of lymphinvasation may delay or prevent clinical disease permanently (Aucouturier, 2002). It has been demonstrated that some drugs effectively prevent the propagation of prion in experimental systems. These include Congo red and its analogs (Caspi, 1998), anthracyclines, amphotericin B and analogs, and tetrapyrroles. These can delay the incubation times of scrapie-infected animals. However, they have toxic effects (Tagliavini, 1997; Mangé, 2000). In tissue culture studies, it has been shown that acridine and phenothiazine compounds (such as quinacrine, and chlorpromazine) used as antimalarials and antipsychotics can inhibit the conversion of PrPC to PrPSc.In animal models, some sulfated sugar polymers, such as pentosan polysulfate, were found to exhibit anti-prion activity. None of these compounds showed activity after the onset of symptoms (Korth, 2001). It increased survival time by approximately 70% when administered between infection and symptom onset. Furthermore, prion titers are usually elevated in the brain during a clinically silent incubation phase, and the rate of prion accumulation determines the onset of symptoms. Therefore, it is thought that treatments that inhibit prion replication can be used prophylactically. Apart from this, the importance of PrP in prion disease is well known, and applications to reduce natural PrP may have a protective effect (Vallabh, 2020). It is also thought that single-stranded antisense oligonucleotides (ASOs) reducing PrP levels may be a new therapeutic option. It is hypothesized that it can reduce the amounts of encoded protein by explicitly binding to the target RNA (Bennett, 2017). The latest approaches include chelation therapy. D-penicillamine, which selectively chelates copper, has been shown to delay the onset of prion disease in animal experiments (Sigurdsson, 2003). An additional beneficial therapeutic approach may also be immunological. Immunization with alpha-helical peptides may successfully reduce cerebral amyloid deposition, a crucial neuropathological feature in Alzheimer's disease (Sigurdsson, 2006).

Conclusion

Currently, there is no effective treatment method. However, a better understanding of the pathogenesis will enable the implementation of effective therapeutic interventions shortly.

References

Abu-Rumeileh, S., Redaelli, V., Baiardi, S., Mackenzie, G., Windl, O., Ritchie, D. L, Parchi, P. (2018). Sporadic fatal insomnia in Europe: phenotypic features and diagnostic challenges. *Annals of Neurology, 84*(3), 347-360. https://doi.org/10.1002/ana.25300.

Aucouturier, P., & Carnaud, C. (2002). The immune system and prion diseases: a relationship of complicity and blindness. *Journal of leukocyte biology, 72*(6), 1075-1083. https://doi.org/10.1189/jlb.72.6.1075.

Bennett, C. F., Baker, B. F., Pham, N., Swayze, E., & Geary, R. S. (2017). Pharmacology of antisense drugs. *Annual review of pharmacology and toxicology, 57*, 81-105. https://doi.org/10.1146/annurev-pharmtox-010716-104846.

Bizzi, A., Pascuzzo, R., Blevins, J., Grisoli, M., Lodi, R., Moscatelli, M. E. M., Castelli, G., Cohen, M. L., Schonberger, L. B., Foutz, A., Safar, J. G., Appleby, B. S., & Gambetti, P. (2020). Evaluation of a New Criterion for Detecting Prion Disease with Diffusion Magnetic Resonance Imaging. *JAMA neurology*, 77(9), 1141–1149. https://doi.org/10.1001/jamaneurol.2020.1319.

Budka, H., Aguzzi, A., Brown, P., Brucher, J. M., Bugiani, O., Gullotta, F., Haltia, M., Hauw, J. J., Ironside, J. W., & Jellinger, K. (1995). Neuropathological diagnostic criteria for Creutzfeldt-Jakob disease (CJD) and other human spongiform encephalopathies (prion diseases). *Brain pathology (Zurich, Switzerland*), 5(4), 459–466. https://doi.org/10.1111/j.1750-3639.1995.tb00625.x.

Caspi, S., Halimi, M., Yanai, A., Sasson, S. B., Taraboulos, A., & Gabizon, R. (1998). The anti-prion activity of Congo red: putative mechanism. *Journal of Biological Chemistry, 273*(6), 3484-3489. https://doi.org/10.1074/jbc.273.6.3484.

Cazzaniga, F. A., Bistaffa, E., De Luca, C. M. G., Indaco, A., Bufano, G., Giaccone, G., & Moda, F. (2021). Sporadic Creutzfeldt-Jakob disease: Real-Time Quaking-Induced Conversion (RT-QuIC) assay represents a major diagnostic advance. *European Journal of Histochemistry: EJH, 65*(Suppl 1). https://doi.org/10.4081/ejh.2021.3298.

Chu, M., Xie, K., Zhang, J., Chen, Z., Ghorayeb, I., Rupprecht, S., Wu, L. (2022). Proposal of new diagnostic criteria for fatal familial insomnia. *Journal of neurology, 269*(9), 4909-4919. https://doi.org/10.1007/s00415-022-11135-6.

Forner, S. A., Takada, L. T., Bettcher, B. M., Lobach, I. V., Tartaglia, M. C., Torres-Chae, C., Geschwind, M. D. (2015). Comparing CSF biomarkers and brain MRI in the diagnosis of sporadic Creutzfeldt-Jakob disease. Neurology: *Clinical Practice, 5*(2), 116-125. https://doi.org/10.1212/CPJ.0000000000000011.

Geschwind, M. D., Potter, C. A., Sattavat, M., Garcia, P. A., Rosen, H. J., Miller, B. L., & DeArmond, S. J. (2009). Correlating DWI MRI with pathologic and other features of Jakob-Creutzfeldt disease. *Alzheimer Disease & Associated Disorders, 23*(1), 82-87. https://doi.org/10.1097/wad.0b013e31818323ef.

Geschwind, M. D. (2015). Prion diseases. *Continuum (Minneapolis, Minn.), 21*(6 Neuroinfectious Disease), 1612-38. https://doi.org/10.1212/CON.0000000000000251.

Kim, M. O., Takada, L. T., Wong, K., Forner, S. A., & Geschwind, M. D. (2018). Genetic PrP prion diseases. *Cold Spring Harbor perspectives in biology, 10*(5), a033134. https://doi.org/10.1101/cshperspect.a033134.

Jones, E., Hummerich, H., Viré, E., Uphill, J., Dimitriadis, A., Speedy, H., Campbell, T., Norsworthy, P., Quinn, L., Whitfield, J., Linehan, J., Jaunmuktane, Z., Brandner, S., Jat, P., Nihat, A., How Mok, T., Ahmed, P., Collins, S., Stehmann, C., Sarros, S., Kovacs, G. G., Geschwind, M. D., Golubjatnikov, A., Frontzek, K., Budka, H., Aguzzi, A., Karamujić-Čomić, H., van der Lee, S. J., Ibrahim-Verbaas, C. A., van Duijn, C. M., Sikorska, B., Golanska, E., Liberski, P. P., Calero, M., Calero, O., Sanchez-Juan, P., Salas, A., Martinón-Torres, F., Bouaziz-Amar, E., Haïk, S., Laplanche, J. L., Brandel, J. P., Amouyel, P., Lambert, J. C., Parchi, P., Bartoletti-Stella, A., Capellari, S., Poleggi, A., Ladogana, A., Pocchiari, M., Aneli, S., Matullo, G., Knight, R., Zafar, S., Zerr, I., Booth, S., Coulthart, M. B., Jansen, G. H., Glisic, K., Blevins, J., Gambetti, P., Safar, J., Appleby, B., Collinge, J., & Mead, S. (2020). Identification of novel risk loci and causal insights for sporadic Creutzfeldt-Jakob disease: a genome-wide association study. *The Lancet. Neurology*, 19(10), 840–848. https://doi.org/10.1016/S1474-4422(20)30273-8.

Korth, C., May, B. C., Cohen, F. E., & Prusiner, S. B. (2001). Acridine and phenothiazine derivatives as pharmacotherapeutics for prion disease. *Proceedings of the National Academy of Sciences, 98*(17), 9836-9841. https://doi.org/10.1073/pnas.161274798.

Mangé, A., Nishida, N., Milhavet, O., McMahon, H. E., Casanova, D., & Lehmann, S. (2000). Amphotericin B inhibits the generation of the scrapie isoform of the prion protein in infected cultures. *Journal of virology, 74*(7), 3135-3140. https://doi.org/10.1128/jvi.74.7.3135-3140.2000.

Moda, F., Bolognesi, M. L., & Legname, G. (2019). Novel screening approaches for human prion diseases drug discovery. *Expert Opinion on Drug Discovery, 14*(10), 983-993. https://doi.org/10.1080/17460441.2019.1637851.

Muayqil, T., Gronseth, G., & Camicioli, R. (2012). Evidence-based guideline: diagnostic accuracy of CSF 14-3-3 protein in sporadic Creutzfeldt-Jakob disease: report of the guideline development subcommittee of the American Academy of Neurology. *Neurology, 79*(14), 1499-1506. https://doi.org/10.1212/WNL.0b013e31826d5fc3.

Mundlamurri, R. C., Shah, R., Adiga, M. S., Chatterjee, A., Gautham, B., Raghavendra, K., Sinha, S. (2020). EEG observations in probable sporadic CJD. *Annals of Indian Academy of Neurology, 23*(6), 760. https://doi.org/10.4103/aian.AIAN_672_20.

Paterson, R. W., Torres-Chae, C. C., Kuo, A. L., Ando, T., Nguyen, E. A., Wong, K., Geschwind, M. D. (2012). Differential diagnosis of Jakob-Creutzfeldt disease. *Archives of neurology, 69*(12), 1578-1582. https://doi.org/10.1001/2013.jamaneurol.79.

Prusiner, S. B. (1998). Prions. *Proceedings of the National Academy of Sciences, 95*(23), 13363-13383. https://doi.org/10.1073/pnas.95.23.13363.

Sigurdsson, E. M. (2006). Immunotherapy for conformational diseases. *Current pharmaceutical design, 12*(20), 2569-2585. https://doi.org/10.2174/13816120 6777698837.

Sigurdsson, E. M., Brown, D. R., Alim, M. A., Scholtzova, H., Carp, R., Meeker, H. C., Wisniewski, T. (2003). Copper chelation delays the onset of prion disease. *Journal of Biological Chemistry, 278*(47), 46199-46202. https://doi.org/10.1074/jbc.C300303200.

Sigurdson, C. J., Bartz, J. C., & Glatzel, M. (2019). Cellular and molecular mechanisms of prion disease. *Annual Review of Pathology: Mechanisms of Disease, 14*, 497-516. https://doi.org/10.1146/annurev-pathmechdis-012418-013109.

Takada, L. T., & Geschwind, M. D. (2013, September). Prion diseases. In *Seminars in neurology* (Vol. 33, No. 04, pp. 348-356). Thieme Medical Publishers. https://doi.org/10.1055/s-0033-1359314.

Tagliavini, F., McArthur, R. A., Canciani, B., Giaccone, G., Porro, M., Bugiani, M., Post, C. (1997). Effectiveness of anthracycline against experimental prion disease in Syrian hamsters. *Science, 276*(5315), 1119-1121. https://doi.org/10.1126/science.276.5315.111.

Thompson, A. G., & Mead, S. H. (2019). Fluid biomarkers in the human prion diseases. *Molecular and Cellular Neuroscience, 97*, 81-92. https://doi.org/10.1016/j.mcn.2018.12.003.

Vallabh, S. M., Minikel, E. V., Schreiber, S. L., & Lander, E. S. (2020). Towards a treatment for genetic prion disease: trials and biomarkers. *The Lancet Neurology, 19*(4), 361-368. https://doi.org/10.1016/S1474-4422(19)30403-X.

Zerr, I., Kallenberg, K., Summers, D. M., Romero, C., Taratuto, A., Heinemann, U., Breithaupt, M., Varges, D., Meissner, B., Ladogana, A., Schuur, M., Haik, S., Collins, S. J., Jansen, G. H., Stokin, G. B., Pimentel, J., Hewer, E., Collie, D., Smith, P., Roberts, H., & Sanchez-Juan, P. (2009). Updated clinical diagnostic criteria for sporadic Creutzfeldt-Jakob disease. *Brain:a journal of neurology*, 132(Pt 10), 2659–2668. https://doi.org/10.1093/brain/awp191.

Chapter 17

Congenital Central Nervous System Infections

Mehmet Güçlü*, MD
Department of Obstetrics and Gynecology, Marmara University, Istanbul, Turkiye

Abstract

Congenital infections of the central nervous system can be defined as clinical conditions occurring as a result of short- or long-term adverse impacts of microorganisms transmitted during intrauterine life on the central nervous system. Congenital cytomegalovirus, rubella, toxoplasma, and group B streptococcal infections will be discussed in this chapter. In the viremic or bacteremic phase of the mother infection, these microorganisms can pass from the mother to the fetus through transplacental transmission and exert various effects. Moreover, these pathogens can cross intact fetal membranes during the intrauterine period. Fetal infections may occur in the early stages of pregnancy and cause significant clinical conditions at birth. In another form of transmission (vertical transmission), microorganisms can proliferate and infect the fetus during childbirth through the vagina and cervix. There is strong evidence between the resulting brain damage and the infant's exposure to perinatal infection and inflammation. The general view is that an initiating event causes a maternal or fetal inflammatory response, which ultimately contributes to adverse outcomes such as intraventricular hemorrhage, white matter damage, and neurodevelopmental disabilities (cerebral palsy). All these adverse outcomes can be reduced with some protective measures. Hence, mothers must be screened for infections before and during pregnancy and, if possible, immunization should be performed before pregnancy. If it is impossible, contagiousness should be reduced with some precautions at birth. It is possible to reduce the

* Corresponding Author's Email: drmguclu@gmail.com.

In: Central Nervous System Infections
Editor: Mustafa Usanmaz
ISBN: 979-8-89113-660-1

possibility of transmission of some infections by drug treatments applied to the mother or the infant.

Keywords: rubella, cytomegalovirus, group B streptococcal infection, toxoplasmosis

Introduction

Viral and bacterial infections can cause serious problems in the fetus and newborn by infecting the fetus during pregnancy or childbirth. In a healthy adult, the said infections may cause asymptomatic or only mild non-specific symptoms. Then, the microorganisms may lie dormant for a long time and cause various clinical conditions, such as shedding of asymptomatic virus. There is decreased maternal cell-dependent immunity to viral infections during pregnancy. Hence, pregnant women and their fetuses are theoretically at a higher risk of disease. Depending on the week of gestation, transplacental viral infection can cause changes from asymptomatic to fetal or neonatal death or long-term sequelae. Prevention seems to be the leading method in the management of diseases due to insufficient specific antiviral treatment opportunities in newborns and fetuses. Congenital infection that develops as a result of neonatal group B streptococcal colonization occurs when microorganisms pass through the birth canal of the colonized mother. Infection can be reduced by screening for this colonization with appropriate cultures to be taken during pregnancy and applying antibiotic prophylaxis to pregnant women with positive culture results during childbirth. As a result of antibody screening for measles before pregnancy, the vaccination of expectant mothers with insufficient immunity will reduce the possibility of transmission of this infection.

Cytomegalovirus Infection

Cytomegalovirus (CMV) represents a DNA virus from the Herpes virus family that can cause multiple infection syndromes in people. Furthermore, most CMV infections in humans remain undetected because of their high rate of quiescent effect on the host. Additionally, the mentioned virus can cause intrauterine and neonatal infections. About 10% of healthy adults develop a syndrome with fever, atypical lymphocytosis, malaise, and lymphadenopathy when first infected with CMV. The virus can be excreted in tears, breast milk, cervical secretions, and urine for weeks, months, or years after primary infection. The latent period occurs eventually, but reinfection and reactivation are frequent (Raynor, 1993). About 50% of women of reproductive age have antibodies to CMV. A significant increase in titration usually indicates primary infection. Immunoglobulin M can be detected four to eight weeks after primary infection. However, the elevation may be periosteal or remain low for years. The best results for tests used to detect congenital CMV infection in amniotic fluid samples are acquired after amniocentesis after 21 weeks of gestation and at least six weeks after the initial diagnosis of maternal infection (Enders et al., 2001; Liesnard et al., 2000). The fetus may be infected through transplacental transmission or exposure to the virus through the birth canal or cervix. The serological or culture evaluation findings of intrauterine CMV infection are observed in 0.2-2.2% of all live births (Griffiths et al., 1980).

Contrary to other viral infections, CMV can infect the newborn or fetus despite the presence of maternal antibodies due to its intermittent excretion and latency through the female genital tract. The cervical excretion of the virus increases with the progression of pregnancy, and the infection rate is higher in infants born to mothers with virus shedding. The most severe neonatal infection is observed in infants born to mothers who have had a primary infection during pregnancy (Enders et al., 2001; Liesnard et al., 2000). Approximately 1% of all newborns have cytomegalovirus. Approximately 5-10% of newborns born infected are clinically asymptomatic at birth. The virus in question causes cytomegalic inclusion disease. In this syndrome low birth weight, microcephaly, intracranial calcifications, chorioretinitis, mental and motor retardation, sensorineural deficits, hepatosplenomegaly, jaundice, hemolytic anemia, and thrombocytopenic purpura develop. Congenital sensorineural hearing loss is the most common finding in newborns born symptomatic at a rate of 30% (Hicks et al., 1993). Microcephaly, which is frequently associated with paraventricular cerebral calcification, is also quite common (Ahlfors et al., 1986). Although the complete eradication of the virus seems possible, the formation of antibodies after primary infection in people can reduce the rates of congenital fetal infection and related sequelae. Thus, it is clear that the prevention of maternal infection is the main strategy to prevent intrauterine infection. Recommendations should be made on the serological screening of women in the high-risk group and the taking of hygiene measures by suspicious individuals. Although the complete eradication of the virus is impossible, the formation of antibodies after primary infection in people can reduce the rates of congenital fetal infection and related sequelae. Hence, effective CMV vaccination will be considered a significant advance.

Rubella Infection

Measles represents a highly infectious disease of the paramyxovirus family, affecting children mostly. Most adults are immune to measles. However, when measles becomes an epidemic, pneumonia can develop in unvaccinated women. Accordingly, negative outcomes can be observed in the mother and fetus (Eberhart-Phillips et al., 1993; Stein and Greenspoon, 1991). The clinical diagnosis of measles is established based on a maculopapular rash, photophobia, and upper respiratory tract symptoms emerging one to two days after specific exant hematous rashes (Koplik patches). A definitive diagnosis can be established with serological tests. Subacute sclerosing panencephalitis (SSPE) is a chronic infection of the central nervous system that occurs at the end of a latent period of one to ten years following a measles infection. The first signs and symptoms emerge years after exposure to the measles virus, with an average of seven to eight years of age being the period when it is most commonly observed. Behavioral changes, myoclonus, visual disturbances, and pyramidal and extrapyramidal symptoms are among the first signs of the disease. The disease usually results in death within 1-3 years. SSPE can be observed in the form of late cases, particularly in relation to hormonal and immune system changes during pregnancy (Wirguin et al., 1988). In congenital measles, rashes can be observed in the infant at birth and in a ten-day period. Sometimes, the measles virus can be transmitted from the mother through the placenta in an amount that does not need replication and can cause disease, and it can cause simultaneous disease in the mother and child. Children of mothers who have been vaccinated against measles in childhood, but whose measles antibody titers have decreased during pregnancy, pose a risk of measles transmission and SSPE in the first six months. Since there is no effective treatment for SSPE, the significance of regular implementation of vaccination programs in childhood, adolescence, and adulthood should be stressed. Serological screening of women for vaccine-preventable diseases, involving measles, before pregnancy, vaccination against infections to which they are not immune, and becoming pregnant in an appropriate period after vaccination will contribute significantly to decreasing the incidence of rare diseases in communities.

Group B Streptococcal Infections

Group B streptococci (GBS) have recently been among the most important causes of neonatal infection and are now accepted as one of the leading causes of neonatal morbidity and mortality. Group B streptococci can be isolated from the vagina and cervix at a rate of 10%-30% in any period of pregnancy (Regan et al., 1996). Colonization can be temporary, chronic, or intermittent. Vaginal and cervical contamination and colonization are considered to be of gastrointestinal origin. Between 3% and 12% of all newborns in total are colonized with GBS during their first week of life. Vertical transmission is observed at a higher rate when the maternal carriage is localized to the cervix compared to rectal localization. In recent years, GBS has become the most significant cause of septicemia and meningitis in the newborn's first three months. Newborns with GBS infection have two distinct clinical syndromes. The first clinical syndrome is an early-onset infection, which occurs in the first seven days of life and accounts for almost three-quarters of cases in infants younger than three months. Approximately 72% of these cases occur in the first 24 hours of life. A significant part of these infections presents with symptoms either at birth or in the first 90 minutes after birth, which indicates that GBS exposure and infection occur frequently in utero. Whereas the incidence is 1.8 per 100 live births in the normal population, this rate ranges from ten to 60 in infants of maternal GBS carriers. It is estimated that early neonatal infection occurs as a result of vertical transmission from a mother colonized with GBS. In a study conducted, this disease emerged as bacteremia (80%), pneumonia (7%), and meningitis (6%). Of these cases, 83% are preterm newborns (Schrag et al., 2000). The second type of infection (late-onset) occurs from the first week of life to the third month of life. Although it is thought that some infants are colonized at birth and subsequently develop invasive diseases, the nosocomial transmission may be as important as vertical transmission. The late-onset disease mostly occurs as bacteremia (63%), but it also occurs as meningitis (24%). Approximately 50% of meningitis survivors will develop neurologic sequelae, e.g., cortical blindness, diabetes insipidus, deafness, and other cranial nerve defects and spasticity. According to the culture-based approach to prevent neonatal infection, all women are screened for group B streptococcal colonization at 35 to 37 weeks of gestation. Accordingly, antibiotics are administered to the carriers during the intrapartum period. Ampicillin is a commonly used drug, and clindamycin or erythromycin can be used in individuals allergic to penicillin.

Toxoplasma Infection

The obligate intracellular parasite, Toxoplasma gondii, causes toxoplasmosis. Unless pregnancy is present, the infection is generally subclinical and harmless in immunocompetent individuals; however, vertical transmission can occur during pregnancy. Toxoplasmosis is transmitted to humans in three main ways. It is estimated that about 50% of cases in the United States of America occur after ingesting undercooked meat containing tissue cysts (Dubey, 1994; Roghmann et al., 1999). The second way of contracting toxoplasmosis may be in the form of oral ingestion of oocytes in the environment from cat litter boxes with contaminated cat feces, from the infected soil, or as a result of eating vegetables and fruits that have contacted the contaminated soil without washing them. The third mode of transmission is transplacental transmission, which occurs when primary infection develops during pregnancy (Jones et al., 2001). Since acute toxoplasma infections are relatively asymptomatic, a common problem for obstetricians is how to detect acute infection during pregnancy. Although screening is frequently discussed in the United States of America, it is not generally implemented in practice. It may be challenging to interpret serological tests conducted for diagnostic purposes, and PCR and ultrasound in the amniotic fluid are other beneficial diagnostic methods. Ultrasound findings are non-specific, but ventricular dilatation (most common), intracranial calcification, increased placental thickness, liver enlargement, and ascites are observed in more than 1/3 of cases with fetal infection (Daffos et al., 1988).

Immunocompetent pregnant women have a minimal risk of maternal toxoplasmosis, and 90% of infections in these individuals are asymptomatic and self-limiting. Symptoms may be in the form of axillary or posterior cervical lymphadenopathy, fatigue, and muscle aches. On the other hand, fetal risks vary considerably and change according to the trimester when the disease is acquired and the presence and absence of maternal treatment. If maternal seroconversion occurs at or before the 5th week of gestation, there is no or very low risk of fetal infection; however, if seroconversion occurs in the third trimester, up to 60% of newborns may develop congenital infection (Forestier et al., 1991). Subclinical infection present in up to 85% of newborns will manifest itself later as growth retardation, hearing loss, and chorioretinitis. The frequency of severe sequelae, such as intrauterine death, neurological disorders, hydrocephalus, cerebral calcification, and severe vision loss, at or after birth, can be reduced by prenatal antibiotic treatment without changing the rate of congenital infection (Gilbert et al., 2001). It should be accepted that pregnant women with IgG positivity at the beginning of pregnancy are at low risk for congenital infection that will occur later. Preventing acute infection during pregnancy should be preferred. Particularly pregnant women with negative IgG should be informed about the precautions to be taken during pregnancy. When maternal infection is detected, spiramycin treatment should be started immediately, and if the amniotic fluid PCR analysis is found in favor of fetal infection, pyrimycin/sulfadiazine should be added to the treatment.

Conclusion

Transpasental and vertical transmission are the two most important ways of transmission of microorganisms causing congenital CNS infections from the mother to the fetus. This transmission and the possibility of disease can be reduced with some precautions to be taken by the mother. These can be achieved successfully with options such as pre-pregnancy vaccination for measles and intrapartum antibiotic prophylaxis for Group B streptococci. Hence, all women must be screened for measles antibodies before pregnancy, and those without immunity must be vaccinated. During pregnancy, cultures should be taken for group B streptococcal screening between 35 and 37 weeks in line with the protocols, and antibiotic prophylaxis should be applied to pregnant women with growth in culture. Prevention measures should be paid attention to during pregnancy for toxoplasmosis, and prenatal antibiotic treatment should be considered to reduce severe neonatal sequelae. There is currently no accepted treatment modality for treating acute maternal or neonatal infection caused by CMV.

References

Ahlfors, K., Ivarsson, S. A., & Bjerre, I. (1986). Microcephaly and congenital cytomegalovirus infection: a combined prospective and retrospective study of a Swedish infant population. *Pediatrics*, *78*(6), 1058-1063.https://doi.org/10.1542/peds.78.6.1058.

Daffos, F., Forestier, F., Capella-Pavlovsky, M., Thulliez, P., Aufrant, C., Valenti, D., & Cox, W. L. (1988). Prenatal management of 746 pregnanciesat risk for congenital toxoplasmosis. *New England Journal of Medicine,318*, 271-275. https://doi.org/10.1056/NEJM198802043180502.

Dubey, J. P. (1994). Toxoplasmosis. *Journal of the American Veterinary Medical Association,* 205, 1593-1598.

Eberhart-Phillips, J. E., Frederick, P. D., Baron, R. C., & Mascola, L. (1993). Measles in pregnancy: a descriptive study of 58 cases. *Obstetrics and Gynecology*, *82*(5), 797-801.

Enders, G., Bäder, U., Lindemann, L., Schalasta, G., & Daiminger, A. (2001). Prenatal diagnosis of congenital cytomegalovirus infection in 189 pregnancies with known outcome. *Prenataldiagnosis*, *21*(5), 362-377. https://doi.org/10.1002/pd.59.

Forestier, F., Daffos, F., Hohlfeld, P., & Lynch L. (1991). Infectious fetal diseases. Prevention, prenatal diagnosis, practical measures. *Presse Medicale, 20,* 1448-1454.

Gilbert, R. E., Gras, L., Wallon, M., Peyron, F., Ades, A. E., & Dunn, D. T. (2001). Effect of prenatal treatment on mother to child transmission of Toxoplasma gondii: retrospective cohort study of 554 mother-child pairs in Lyon, France. *International Journal of Epidemiology, 30,* 1303-1308.

Griffiths, P. D., Campbell-Benzie, A., & Heath, R. B. (1980). A prospective study of primary cytomegalovirus infection in pregnant women. *BJOG: An International Journal of Obstetrics & Gynaecology*, *87*(4), 308-314.

Hicks, T., Fowler, K., Richardson, M., Dahle, A., Adams, L., & Pass, R. (1993). Congenital cytomegalovirus infection and neonatal auditory screening. *The Journal of Pediatrics*, *123*(5), 779-782. https://doi.org/10.1016/S0022-3476(05)80859-5.

Jones, J. L., Lopez, A., Wilson, M., Schulkin, J., & Gibbs, R. (2001). Congenital toxoplasmosis: A review. *Obstetrical and Gynecological survey,56*, 296-305.

Liesnard, C., Donner, C., Brancart, F., Gosselin, F., Delforge, M. L., & Rodesch, F. (2000). Prenatal diagnosis of congenital cytomegalovirus infection: prospective study of 237 pregnancies at risk. *Obstetrics & Gynecology*, *95*(6), 881-888. https://doi.org/10.1016/S0029-7844(99)00657-2.

Raynor, B. D. (1993). Cytomegalovirus infection in pregnancy. *Seminars in perinatology*, *17*(6), 394-402.

Regan, J. A., Klebanoff, M. A., Nugent, R. P., Eschenbach, D. A., Blackwelder, W. C., Lou, Y., Gibbs, R. S. Petting, P. J., Martin, D. H., Edelman, R., & VIP Study Group. (1996). Colonization with group B streptococci in pregnancy and adverse outcome. *American journal of obstetrics and gynecology*, *174*(4), 1354-1360. https://doi.org/10.1016/S0002-9378(96)70684-1.

Remington, J. S., & Klein, J. O. (2001). *Infectious Diseases of the Fetus and Newborn Infant* (5th ed). Philadelphia:WB Saunders.

Roghmann, M. C., Faulkner, C. T., Lefkowitz A., Patton S., Zimmermann J., Morris, J. G. (1999).Decreased seroprevalence for Toxoplasma gondii in Seventh Day Adventists in Maryland. *The American Journal of Tropical Medicine and Hygiene, 60*(5), 790-792.https://doi.org/10.4269/ajtmh.1999.60.790.

Schrag, S. J., Zywicki, S., Farley, M. M., Reingold, A. L., Harrison, L. H., Lefkowitz, L. B., Hadler, J. L., Danila, R., Cieslak, P. R., & Schuchat, A. (2000). Group B streptococcal disease in the era of intrapartum antibiotic prophylaxis. *New England Journal of Medicine*, *342*(1), 15-20. https://doi.org/10.1056/NEJM200001063420103.

R

S

T

V

W